Fundamentals of Diagnosing and Treating Eating Disorders

Janna Gordon-Elliott

Fundamentals of Diagnosing and Treating Eating Disorders

A Clinical Casebook

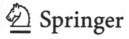
Springer

Janna Gordon-Elliott
New York, NY
USA

ISBN 978-3-319-46063-5   ISBN 978-3-319-46065-9   (eBook)
DOI 10.1007/978-3-319-46065-9

Library of Congress Control Number: 2016950904

Printed on acid-free paper

This Springer imprint is published by Springer Nature
The registered company is Springer International Publishing AG
The registered company address is: Gewerbestrasse 11, 6330 Cham, Switzerland

Preface

Epitomized by the prototypical disorders of anorexia nervosa and bulimia nervosa, *feeding and eating disorders* span a wide range of disturbance related to eating, weight regulation, and body image, and impact individuals across gender, sexual orientation, racial/ethnic, and socioeconomic lines. It has been estimated that up to 20 million women and 10 million men in the USA may be affected by a clinically significant eating disorder at some point in their lives, and many more will have sub-syndromal disturbances in eating, body image, and weight concerns [1]. The impact of feeding and eating disorders is substantial, with significant medical, psychological, and functional consequences. Anorexia nervosa, for example, appears to carry the highest mortality rate of all psychiatric disorders, and the long-term physical, emotional, and social sequelae add to further burden—for the individual and society.

The high prevalence and pernicious impact of full-syndrome feeding and eating disorders as well as subclinical troubles in eating and body image should prompt careful attention to the possible presence of eating-disordered symptoms in all patients in clinical practice, whether or not issues of eating or weight are part of the chief complaint. Moreover, feeding and eating disorders may coexist with other mental and medical conditions or may manifest

in atypical ways. Mental health clinicians and practitioners across clinical specialties and disciplines will benefit from additional knowledge and skills related to the recognition and initial management of feeding and eating disorders. With enhanced detection, assessment, and appropriate referral, more individuals struggling with problematic eating patterns or ideas about body or weight may have the benefit of treatment.

Many changes were made in the categorization and diagnosis of eating disorders with the transition of the Diagnostic and Statistical Manual (DSM) from DSM-IV-TR to DSM-5, including combining diagnoses from different chapters and revising the diagnostic criteria of others.

In this book, illustrative cases are utilized to demonstrate the eight feeding and eating disorders, in addition to a range of presentations that are not clearly as "typical" but which still may be common in clinical practice. Changes in DSM-5 affecting the feeding and eating disorders are reviewed. Strategies and clinical pearls related to the recognition, assessment, and management of eating disorder pathology in patients in clinical practice are discussed through the viewpoint of vivid case presentations.

Clinical material is drawn from the author's clinical work with patients over years and in different treatment settings, as well as idealized and prototypical diagnostic presentations. All cases presented have been developed by the author combining characteristics of real individuals as well as fictitious elements. No case presented represents a specific individual. First names were created and assigned alphabetically and have no connection to actual patients.

New York, USA   Janna Gordon-Elliott

References

1. American Psychiatric Association. (2013). *Diagnostic and statistical manual of mental disorders* (5th ed.). Arlington, VA: American Psychiatric Publishing.
2. Wade TD, Keski-Rahkonen A, & Hudson J. (2011). Epidemiology of eating disorders. In M. Tsuang and M. Tohen (Eds.), *Textbook in Psychiatric Epidemiology* (3rd ed.) (pp. 343–360). New York: Wiley.

Contents

Part I
Patients who Eat Too Little

Part I
Patients Who Die Too Late

Chapter 1
Arlene, an Anxious Young Woman

1.1 Case Presentation

Arlene is a 22-year-old woman who is coming for a first appointment with a psychiatrist, Dr. Bond, with a chief complaint of "anxiety." Arlene graduated from small, elite college in the North East six months prior and has been living with her parents since then, interning in a law office, while studying for the Law School Admission Test (LSAT). Her father made the appointment to see the psychiatrist due to concerns that she seems more withdrawn than usual. He told Dr. Bond over the phone, while making the appointment, that he and his wife are worried that she seems sad and withdrawn, and that she has been losing weight. He asks to come in to talk with Dr. Bond before Arlene's first appointment, but Dr. Bond suggests that he meet with Arlene on her own, to which her father reluctantly agrees.

Arlene presents as a thin young woman wearing a loose-fitting sweater, tailored slacks, and dress shoes. She has a large backpack and a yoga mat with her, with a large water bottle in the side pocket of her bag. She explains that her parents have asked her to come in because they think she is not the "superstar they think I'm supposed to be," but that she is willing to be here as it might be helpful to talk. She reports that she has been working long hours in the law

© Springer International Publishing Switzerland 2017
J. Gordon-Elliott, *Fundamentals of Diagnosing and Treating Eating Disorders*, DOI 10.1007/978-3-319-46065-9_1

firm, returning home after 10 pm most nights, eating dinner on her own, and waking up early to go for a run "to relax" before going to work at 8:30 am. She has several friends from high school and college in the area, but she says that she has been tending to stay to herself, spending weekends studying in coffee shops in the neighborhood, taking walks, or going to yoga classes. She feels like she needs this "solitude" in order to get her LSAT preparation in and cope with the stress of her workplace. She describes feeling tired much of the time, attributing this to her work schedule and "having to wake up early" in order to run, though also describes having a lot of "nervous energy," which is why she likes to walk home from the firm and stay active. She acknowledges that her concentration does not seem to be as good as it had been in high school and college, though believes that this is due to the under-stimulating content involved in studying for the LSAT compared to school coursework. She denies feeling depressed and denies suicidal ideation.

Elaborating on her earlier comment about her parents' expectations, she explains that she was always an "overachiever," at the top of her class in high school and for much of college; her extracurricular activities as a child included playing the viola, performing with an orchestra in numerous high-profile local concerts. She was otherwise a "quiet" child. She had a few good friends and was well liked by teachers and classmates. She describes always having felt "a little out of place" among her peers, with anxiety in some social contexts, feeling she was never sure what others' "really thought" about her.

Regarding her eating and weight, she admits that she has been eating "less" since returning home and that she has lost "some weight" but denies knowing what her weight had been at the time of graduation. She reports that she is vegetarian but does not spontaneously give more information about her diet. She relates, with further questioning, that she was always "pretty slim," though had gained some weight in late high school and the first year of college. She admits that in her junior year of college she lost "a lot" of weight in a fairly short period of time, explaining that she had been sick with a gastroenteritis and had lost 2 or 3 lb, and upon recovering, continued to make an effort to limit her food intake, finding it "interesting to experiment" with eating very little. She says that this went on for about one month, with her weight loss

noticeable to others. Her grades dipped and she was feeling very tired all the time. She began eating more normally after that, though continued to avoid meat (which she had done for the first time during this period) and to eat less than she had been eating before the episode.

She denies wanting to lose weight or "be stick thin," but is noticeably more clipped in her responses when Dr. Bond asks questions on this topic and about the specifics of what she eats. She agrees to return for another appointment the following week.

1.2 Diagnosis/Assessment

Preferred diagnosis: anorexia nervosa

Arlene most likely has a diagnosis of anorexia nervosa (AN). Individuals with AN restrict food, maintaining a low weight, with a disturbed experience of body image or lack of insight into the seriousness of the low weight. Those who, in addition to restricting food, also compensate for food intake through vomiting or laxative use (whether or not they binge eat), fall under the *Binge-eating/purging* type; all others are classified as *restricting* type [see Text Box: Anorexia Nervosa: DSM-5 Diagnostic Criteria].

Anorexia Nervosa: DSM-5 Diagnostic Criteria

A. Restriction of energy intake relative to requirements, leading to a significantly low body weight in the context of age, sex, developmental trajectory, and physical health.

B. Intense fear of gaining weight or of becoming fat, or persistent behavior that interferes with weight gain, even though at a significantly low weight.

C. Disturbance in the way in which one's body weight or shape is experienced, undue influence of body weight or shape on self-evaluation, or persistent lack of recognition of the seriousness of the current low body weight.

Subtypes:

Restricting type

Binge-eating/purging type

Specify if:
   In partial remission
   In full remission
Specify current severity:
   Mild: BMI > 17
   Moderate: BMI 16–16.99
   Severe: BMI 15–15.99
   Extreme: BMI < 15

Over time working with Arlene, both during her illness and recovery, Dr. Bond learned more about the quality of her symptoms and the course of her illness. She has lost 20 lb over the six months before presenting to see him for the first time, weighing 98 lbs at 5 foot 6 in. tall, with a resulting decline in her body mass index (BMI) from 19 to 15.8 [see the text box on Body Mass Index (BMI) in Chap. 12]. She had cut back her overall calorie intake substantially, was eating a more restricted range of foods, and had developed limited flexibility in terms of what she eats for each meal. She would become acutely distressed (tearful and angry) when her meal plan was altered due to external factors (such as dinner out with others, or any unexpected change in her routine that makes her unable to have her planned meal). She knew she was very thin and getting thinner (to a degree that at times she knew might be worrisome), but became upset whenever she imagined loosening up her food restrictions or decreasing her exercise, and then gaining weight.

She had become increasingly preoccupied with food despite eating much less—spending time in the kitchen organizing the fridge, cleaning the dishes and countertops, reading about food and nutrition, and offering food to others. In his study of induced starvation in a group of healthy male controls in the mid-1940s, researcher Ancel Keys documented changes exceedingly similar to some of the core features of AN, including depression and emotional instability, social isolation, preoccupation with food (including thinking about food, hoarding food, even during the "recovery" period where food was no longer restricted), and self-reported impairment in concentration and other cognitive capacities, indicating that many of the psychological and cognitive signs and symptoms of AN may be a direct effect of starvation,

itself, regardless of whether it is self-imposed or what the underlying motivations for food restriction are.

After partial recovery, Arlene was able to report that her concentration had become very poor and she was having difficulty
focusing on her studying. In addition, her sleep had become more
fitful—and despite feeling tired most of the time, she had a restless
energy that would keep her up at night and that often prompted her
to keep moving (taking walks outside, pacing in her room). The
excessive activity that patients with AN exhibit may have multiple
causes; in addition to a conscious effort to move in order to burn
calories, changes in neuropeptides related to starvation appear to
directly effect activity level and sleep leading to motor restlessness
as well as changes in sleep duration and architecture.

Other physiologic changes that are well documented in AN
include a decrease in basal metabolic rate and resting heart rate,
hypotension, hypothermia, dry skin, brittle hair and hair loss, and
growth of lanugo (fine, unpigmented hair all over body).
Laboratory abnormalities may include hyponatremia and hypokalemia, hypercholesterolemia, elevated liver enzymes, thyroid dysfunction, low estrogen and low testosterone. Patients with AN
experience a loss of bone density and may develop osteoporosis.
Female AN patients may stop menstruating (girls who have not yet
reached menarche may experience a halting of maturation of secondary sexual characteristics and onset of menses). Cardiac
hypotrophy may be found; arrhythmias may develop due to electrolyte disturbances or as a consequence of structural changes in
the heart. Cerebral atrophy has also been identified in individuals
with AN. Individuals with AN who vomit to purge food or misuse
laxatives will be at risk for the metabolic and physiologic consequences related to these behaviors [see Chap. 7].

Behavioral changes that are seen in AN include highly rou-
tinized and restricted eating patterns, with a significantly reduced
range of "allowable" foods and a need to eat the same things every
day (at the same time and under the same circumstances). There is
increased intake of non- or low-nutritive foods, such as water,
zero-calorie drinks, and low-calorie foods; a general shift develops
toward low-density food choices, with a decrease in percent of
calories coming from fat. Individuals with AN may exercise
excessively as a way of expending more calories, or engage in
other compensatory behaviors such as vomiting or laxative use [see

Chap. 5 for further discussion of athletes and eating disorders; see Chap. 7 for discussion of compensatory behaviors and bulimia nervosa]. They may become socially isolative, in part as a way of maintaining extreme control over their eating and behavior, though a restricted range of interests other than food and body may develop that in turn lowers inherent motivation to engage in previously enjoyable activities and social situations. Some individuals may look to "guidance" on lowering weight or maintaining a very low weight; in more recent times, there has been an increase in the use of Internet sites and social media for such purposes, and there has been a concerning emergence of arguably malignant sites that promote unhealthy and dangerous behaviors and body ideals [see Chap. 6 for further discussion].

Predisposing factors that may be related to the development of AN include perfectionistic traits and a family history of an eating disorder. There have been many theories of particular family dynamics that may predispose to AN, though there is substantial variation across patients and these speculations have not been objectively proven. An initial small loss of weight—perhaps, for example, due to an attempt at "dieting" or a gastrointestinal infection—may serve as an initial trigger in a susceptible individual. Progressive conscious control over food intake and energy expenditure may then occur to perpetuate the weight loss; with time, the effects of starvation may contribute to the rigid behavioral control and cognitive distortions that perpetuate the illness.

Spotlight on DSM-5: anorexia nervosa

The diagnostic criteria for AN that changed from DSM-IV-TR to DSM-5 include adjustment of the language regarding the patient's weight, itself (DSM-5 eliminated any reference to percent of "expected" body weight), replacing this with a more general statement that weight must be "significantly" low; elimination of the amenorrhea criterion, as this was not found to add to the validity of the diagnosis and could not be applied to males or prepubescent females; and modifications in the way the motivation for weight loss is described, expanding the criteria to include individuals who might not readily demonstrate body image distortion or who are consciously "refusing" food, but who are—in their behavior—not permitting maintenance of a healthy weight.

1.3 Differential Diagnosis

The differential diagnosis for Arlene is broad—even broader when one considers all patients with symptoms suggestive of AN. In his evaluation, Dr. Bond would want to assess for a depressive illness, such as major depressive disorder, and Anxiety Disorders, such as social anxiety disorder or generalized anxiety disorder. Obsessive–compulsive disorder may share qualities with AN and should be ruled out. Other conditions to include in the differential diagnosis for an individual with AN include separation anxiety disorder, personality disorders (obsessive–compulsive personality disorder, avoidant personality disorder may be more common, though "Cluster B" Personality Disorders such as borderline personality disorder may overlap significantly with all eating disorders, including AN [see discussion in Chap. 8]), body dysmorphic disorder [see Chap. 2 for further discussion], and other feeding and eating disorders.

> **Focus on Differential Diagnosis**
> What distinguishes this case (and AN, in general) from bulimia is, most notably, the emphasis on low weight, itself, rather than the eating behaviors. While a patient with AN may engage in some degree of binging and compensatory behaviors, the most salient aspects of the presentation should include maintenance of a "significantly" low weight and distorted body image and/or impaired insight into the seriousness of the low weight. The other feeding and eating disorder to consider in a very low weight individual is avoidant–restrictive food intake disorder (ARFID). In ARFID, the speculated cause of weight loss and dysfunctional eating should not be a desire for thinness or a distorted body image [see Chap. 4].

AN carries a high mortality risk, perhaps the highest of all psychiatric disorders—a combination of the medical effects of starvation and an elevated suicide risk (with some studies documenting a 25 % lifetime prevalence of suicide attempts in patients with AN). Despite its being a "self-imposed" psychiatric disorder, AN should be considered a potentially fatal illness and addressed with corresponding attention and concern.

The treatment of AN will depend upon the severity of illness. Guidelines have been suggested to help clinicians decide whether a patient needs to be medically hospitalized before being able to be managed as an outpatient, including specific parameters around vital signs, electrocardiogram findings, and laboratory studies. The initial stage of treatment often focuses on refeeding, at least in individuals of markedly low weight. Often this requires an inpatient setting. This may start on a medical service, perhaps even with forced feeds involving a nasogastric feeding tube, with close monitoring for *refeeding syndrome* (characterized by fluid shifts and edema, and metabolic disturbances, including hypophosphatemia, and may be fatal).

Medical hospitalization may be followed by inpatient treatment focusing on the eating disorder, with the emphasis on acclimating the patient to adequate eating behaviors, and working on the psychological factors that precipitated and perpetuated the eating disorder (and which might lead to relapse after recovery). There is evidence for some forms of psychotherapy, including the Maudsley family-based treatment for adolescents with AN, and some forms of Cognitive Behavioral Therapy. There is no clear role for antidepressants, at least very early in the treatment when the individual is very underweight. If there is comorbid depression or an anxiety disorder, initiation of an antidepressant at some point during the recovery period might be useful to address these other conditions that can contribute to eating disorder symptoms. There may also be some utility in antipsychotic medications for anxiolysis related to adapting to a new eating routine, but—in general—no medication is specifically approved for the use in the treatment of AN, and the use of any medication should follow a careful analysis of risks and benefits, and perhaps an expert consultation. Given the increased risk of suicidality in these patients, it is essential that the clinician remains attentive to this, and to ask specifically about suicidal thoughts and behaviors.

The prognosis of AN is variable and guarded. Those receiving aggressive intervention early in their illness may have full and sustained recovery, while those with a longer duration of illness or other factors that complicate their disorder may experience a chronic or relapsing-remitting course. The risk of death, as stated previously, is high, rivaling or exceeding that of the most serious psychiatric disorders.

1.4   Outcome

Arlene was very thin at the time that she was seen by Dr. Bond. She agreed to see her internist for a medical evaluation. Basic blood work demonstrated normal electrolytes; her heart rate was in the low 50 s and her systolic blood pressure was 102; her electrocardiogram was normal other than sinus bradycardia. Based on this workup, her internist and Dr. Bond agreed that it would be adequately safe to continue treatment on an outpatient basis. Over the following several sessions, Dr. Bond was able to engage her about the ways in which her life was currently not meeting her own expectations, and how her eating behaviors might be contributing. Arlene was, with time, able to talk more openly about her concerns about her body, including how she became progressively more preoccupied with her weight and size, weighing herself daily with acute anxiety if the scale went up, and nagging concerns if it stayed the same despite gradually reducing the amount of food she was eating and increasing her walking or the duration of her daily runs. She expressed significant anxiety about many food items which she was sure would immediately "cause the pendulum to swing and make me fat." Referred to a therapist with an expertise in eating disorders, Arlene began a program to address her eating behaviors, with gradual integration of a more variable diet. She was told to limit her exercise, which she initially resisted, but was able to tolerate better with ongoing psychological work. She made efforts to connect more with friends and began finding it easier to feel relaxed with others. Her mood improved. She began talking about how fears about her future had begun feeling very intense as she approached college graduation, and how her focus on her body and food seemed to "solve" this problem, giving her an increased sense of control over her life. As her recovery progressed, she was not found to have any other major psychiatric illness, such as a depressive disorder or anxiety disorder. At stressful junctures of her life in the future, she sometimes found herself considering food restriction as a potential "solution" and remained attentive to not allowing those initial symptoms to progress and take hold of her thinking and behaviors.

Suggested Readings

Frank GK, Shott ME. The role of psychotropic medications in the management of anorexia nervosa: rationale, evidence and future prospects. CNS Drugs. 2016;30(5):419–42.

Shuttleworth E, Sharma S, Lal S, Allan PJ. Medical complications of anorexia nervosa. Br J Hosp Med (Lond). 2016;77(5):287–93.

Zipfel S, Giel KE, Bulik CM, Hay P, Schmidt U. Anorexia nervosa: aetiology, assessment, and treatment. Lancet Psychiatry. 2015;2(12):1099–111.

Chapter 2
Becky's Body Worries

2.1 Case Presentation

Becky is a 29-year-old unmarried woman with asthma and seasonal allergies who is referred to see a psychiatrist, Dr. Clark, by her primary care provider for the evaluation of a possible eating disorder because of expressed preoccupation with what she is eating and a 7 lb weight loss since her last visit six months before. Becky tells Dr. Clark that "this isn't in my head," describing "a rash" on her face which she believes may be related to food allergies. Despite negative allergen testing, she endorses being convinced that she is sensitive to wheat and dairy and that she develops flushing on her face when she eats them. She explains that she has been aware of her flushed skin for the past eight years. Feeling "embarrassed" by this aspect of her appearance, she had tried to manage the symptom on her own for several years, trying numerous topical treatments and home remedies, such as drinking apple cider vinegar. About a year ago, becoming increasingly frustrated by her symptom, she saw a dermatologist who—she reports—told her there was "nothing to see" and seemed "patronizing". Becky saw two more dermatologists after that, whom she describes as equally unresponsive. About two months ago, she began reading about food allergies and is sure that wheat, dairy,

© Springer International Publishing Switzerland 2017   13
J. Gordon-Elliott, *Fundamentals of Diagnosing and Treating Eating Disorders*, DOI 10.1007/978-3-319-46065-9_2

and "nightshade vegetables" are causing her symptoms, so she began progressively limiting her diet. She says the flushing has persisted, but attributes this to her sense that "trace amounts" of these food allergens are present in other foods despite her efforts to buy "pure products". She has been spending an estimated 3 h a day reading about food allergies and checking ingredient lists of foods. She also spends about 2 h in the morning applying makeup to conceal her flushed skin and more time throughout the day when she "checks" on her flushing in her handheld mirror. She avoids looking at herself in bathroom mirrors during the day, afraid of how her flushing might look in "new" mirrors.

Dr. Clark does not appreciate any abnormal discoloration of Becky's skin from her chair across the office room; when she asks where on her face the flushing is, Becky becomes angry, saying that everyone tells her she looks "normal", and the fact that they do not seem to "notice" upsets her even more.

Upon further history, Becky describes a history of worries about her body going back to childhood, with concerns about going blind or dying as a young girl, and worries about the width of her thighs as a teenager. She admits that in high school she would measure her thighs three times a day and do various exercises that she thought might make them smaller. She had a period of food restriction in order to lose weight from her thighs at age 16, reporting that she lost approximately 5 lb over two months but then resumed a more normal diet. She had seen a therapist as an 8-year-olds for her "worries" about sickness and dying; she subsequently saw the school counselor during her senior year because of concerns by her parents and teachers that she was anxious, but she did not find this helpful. She has never been on psychiatric medications.

2.2 Diagnosis/Assessment

Preferred diagnosis: Body Dysmorphic Disorder

With further exploration of her symptoms, Dr. Clark diagnoses Becky with body dysmorphic disorder (BDD). BDD is not considered an eating disorder but has many overlapping features with the feeding and eating disorders and should be considered in the

evaluation of an individual presenting with concerns about physical appearance (see Differential Diagnosis for further discussion).

The diagnosis of BDD requires preoccupations with perceived flaws or defects in one's physical appearance, repetitive behaviors in response to these thoughts about appearance, impairment in functioning due to the preoccupations and behaviors, and the exclusion of an eating disorder that could better explain the patient's symptoms. The individual's physical flaw may not be evident to others; in cases where an objective physical defect is present, the individual's response to the defect surpasses what would be expected, including the intensity of the concerns or the degree of behaviors associated with the defect. Specifiers for BDD include the muscle dysmorphia variant, which applies to individuals focused on not being muscular enough, and the insight specifier (categorized as "with good or fair insight," "with poor insight," and "with absent insight/delusional beliefs"). Previously located in the somatoform disorders section, BDD is currently classified as one of the *obsessive–compulsive and related disorders* in DSM-5, with modifications based on advances in the understanding of the condition [see Text box: "Spotlight on DSM-5: Body Dysmorphic Disorder"].

BDD has a point prevalence of approximately 1.5–2.5, though these estimates are thought to be lower than the actual prevalence, as this diagnosis is often missed—due to various factors, including lack of widespread awareness of, and screening for, the condition, and the shame that individuals with BDD often experience, making them less likely to disclose their thoughts and behaviors about their appearance. In clinical samples, both psychiatric outpatient and inpatient settings, the prevalence is higher; notably, up to one-quarter of all patients seeking non-psychiatric treatment, such as dermatologic and surgical interventions, may have BDD, based on some estimates [2]. BDD is slightly more common in women than men, though this difference is not marked. Gender and cultural standards may influence the focus of the patient's attention; for example, while the most common physical areas of concern include skin, hair, and nose, women with BDD appear to be more preoccupied with weight, breasts, buttock, and legs, while men may be more concerned about their genitals, musculature, and hair/balding.

BDD has a typical age of onset in mid-adolescence and tends to have a chronic course, often taking on different forms over a lifetime (with shifting physical concerns and behaviors). One of the most

important aspects of this condition is its high suicide rate, with suicidal ideation present in as many as 80 % of individuals with BDD and up to 25 % attempting suicide at some point [3].

Treatment, including therapeutic and pharmacologic, can be effective, but relapse rates are high if treatment is not actively continued. Many never receive treatment because they never come to clinical attention (for reasons mentioned previously), or because shame, avoidance, or lack of insight prevents engagement in care. Pharmacologic management of BDD emphasizes serotonin reuptake inhibitors (SRIs, including the selective serotonin reuptake inhibitors, the serotonin norepinephrine reuptake inhibitors, and the tricyclic antidepressants that have potent serotonin reuptake inhibition), often at high doses, with fair response rates but high relapse rates after discontinuation [4]. Antipsychotic medications may sometimes be used to address severe distress or delusional thoughts, though evidence indicates that the delusional variant of BDD is equally responsive to SRIs alone as is the non-delusional type. Relapse rates after a successful treatment with SRIs are very high and therefore might need to be continued long term if not supplemented with another type of treatment, such as Cognitive Behavioral Therapy (CBT). CBT has been demonstrated to be effective for BDD, involving a combination of psychoeducation, challenging the thoughts about appearance that drive the behaviors and distress, and exposure and response prevention (such as looking in the mirror and perceiving flaws, but resisting engaging in maneuvers to hide them). The improvement gained from a treatment course of CBT may endure for an extended period after completion, though there are limited long-term data. An important component of CBT for BDD is relapse prevention, in which the patient might be trained to continue to participate in CBT exercises on his or her own after the therapy is completed, as this seems to improve outcome.

Surgical and other cosmetic treatments to address a patient's perceived flaw is not effective and should not be recommended; BDD symptoms reemerge after these interventions in nearly 100 % of patients. In general, a priority for patients with BDD is detection of the disorder and minimization of iatrogenic harm that might be caused by engaging in repeated treatments and procedures.

It is thought that BDD is substantially more prevalent than population studies indicate, because individuals are not coming to clinical attention. Many patients may be seeking treatment;

however, because of shame related to their concerns and behaviors, or because of clinicians' lack of awareness of BDD or how to detect it, they are not being diagnosed. Experts encourage more broad screening for BDD. The body dysmorphic disorder Questionnaire(BDDQ) is a simple 4-question screening tool, which can be clinician- or patient-administered, and requires no special training to utilize or interpret. It can be found online [http://www.rhodeislandhospital.org/psychiatry/body-image-program.html]; the BDDQ asks about preoccupation with one's appearance and the amount of time and distress that these preoccupations are causing. A positive screen would be an indication for more extensive evaluation, perhaps with an expert.

Spotlight on DSM-5: Body Dysmorphic Disorder

In DSM-III and -IV, BDD was located in the *somatoform disorders* section (the group of diagnoses now referred to as the *somatic symptom disorders*). One major change from DSM-IV to DSM-5 was the development of a new diagnostic category, the *obsessive–compulsive and related disorders*, which includes BDD as well as obsessive–compulsive disorder (OCD) and other disorders, such as Trichotillomania, which appear to share common neurobiological circuitry and have similar clinical phenomenology and response to treatment [1].

The diagnostic criteria for BDD have been modified in DSM-5 to include—in addition to preoccupation with perceived physical flaws or defects—the presence of repetitive thoughts or behaviors in response to the thoughts about physical appearance. In DSM-IV, individuals with beliefs reaching delusional intensity were classified as having *delusional disorder, somatic type*. Emerging evidence, however, indicates that nearly one-half of individuals with BDD may hold their distorted thoughts to a delusional degree and that these individuals do not appear to have significant clinical or demographic differences compared to those with non-delusional beliefs about appearance. The delusional variant may be a more severe form of the illness. DSM-5 added the *absent insight/delusional beliefs* specifier to denote this clinical presentation.

2.3 Differential Diagnosis

Becky presents several different signs and symptoms, including preoccupation with her body both externally (concerns about her skin) and internally (beliefs about the effects certain foods and allergens are causing her); weight loss; anxiety; and ritualistic behaviors. In addition, she has a history of concerns about her body shape leading to food restriction, as well as substantial anxiety symptoms as a youngster. The differential diagnosis is broad, and her evaluation should be thorough.

She was referred for a possible eating disorder. She has experienced recent weight loss. She attributes this to dietary limitations related to her skin; however, individuals with eating disorders will commonly explain their food restriction based on "allergies" or "sensitivities" [see Chap. 14 for further discussion]. To differentiate Becky's presentation from an emerging case of anorexia nervosa (food restriction in an effort to lose weight), Dr. Clark would want to explore the primary motivation for the food limitations as well as Becky's specific concerns about her body. In cases where the preoccupation is primarily about weight or body shape, a diagnosis of an eating disorder should be prioritized. In Becky's case, if the motivation for her food restriction was considered to be for weight loss, but it had not yet led to substantial weight loss, a diagnosis of other specified feeding and eating disorder (not meeting criteria for anorexia nervosa due to weight still within normal limits) would be appropriate. If, on the other hand, she was describing an aversion to certain foods or otherwise refusing to eat them, but not indicating a motivation such as weight loss, then a diagnosis of avoidant–restrictive food intake disorder would be applicable.

Because of ritualistic behavior and intrusive, repetitive thoughts, a diagnosis of OCD should be high in the differential. Indeed, it is thought that there is substantial overlap, neurobiologically and phenomenologically, between OCD and BDD, which led to the categorization change in DSM-5 placing them in the same chapter. In BDD, the focus of the patient's concerns and rituals should be a perceived physical defect or flaw, as opposed to another worry or distress-laden preoccupation (as in the case of OCD).

Other relevant diagnoses include various anxiety disorders, including social anxiety disorder, in which an individual may feel

scrutinized by others; in Becky's case, her specific preoccupation with her skin, and her substantial ritualistic behavior in response to this, would make a diagnosis of BDD more appropriate and useful (for conceptualization and treatment purposes). It is possible that Becky has comorbid generalized anxiety disorder or social anxiety disorder, and this could be further explored. Somatic symptom disorder (known as somatoform disorders prior to DSM-5) should also be considered. In somatic symptom disorder, an individual has significant distress related to physical symptoms. In Becky's case, though she describes flushing and substantial related distress, she is specifically preoccupied with appearance, and thus, the diagnosis of BDD is more apt. Delusional disorder can also be considered. As mentioned previously in this section, delusional variants of BDD were classified as delusional disorder, somatic type prior to DSM-5. As with other alternate diagnoses, Becky's specific focus on a physical appearance-related matter and her associated ritualistic behavior make BDD the most suitable diagnosis.

Individuals with BDD may commonly have comorbid depressive disorders, perhaps in part in response to the distress caused by their physical preoccupation and their ritualistic behaviors. Suicidality, as mentioned previously, is particularly high in this population and should be assessed carefully and in an ongoing way. There may be comorbid anxiety disorders and OCD.

2.4   Outcome

Dr. Clark, after a careful psychiatric evaluation, made a diagnosis of BDD. Becky was initially remained fixated on her appearance flaw and had difficulty considering the possibility that her skin problem was less evident to others than to her. She was resistant to following up with Dr. Clark, insisting that she has a dermatologic or allergic issue; she continued to seek care from other specialists. She denied clear symptoms of a major depressive episode, but did have low mood and reduced concentration; in addition, she felt socially isolated because of her symptoms and her need to spend hours a day doing her rituals. She denied suicidal thoughts. Dr. Clark was able to engage her on the level of the distress that her worries were causing her, and her interpersonal dissatisfaction; she

agreed to follow up with him to "process" some of these feelings. She agreed to try sertraline for her "anxiety and sadness". With time and gentle encouragement, she began to participate with some cognitive restructuring of her body-related thoughts. She started to be more open to the possibility that her distress was at least in part related to BDD. She was eventually referred for a structured course of CBT for BDD with improvement in her overall preoccupation with her skin and the time spent engaging in compensatory behaviors. After several months of seeing Dr. Clark, taking sertraline, and engaging in CBT, Becky was feeling less burdened by her thoughts and her behaviors and was overall happier. She was eating a normal diet, her weight was stable, and she was no longer seeking out medical specialists for her skin.

References

1. Chosak A, Marques L, Greenberg JL, Jenike E, Dougherty DD, Wilhelm S. Body dysmorphic disorder and obsessive-compulsive disorder: similarities, differences and the classification debate. Expert Rev Neurother. 2008;8 (8):1209–18.
2. Fang A, Matheny NL, Wilhelm S. Body dysmorphic disorder. Psychiatr Clin North Am. 2014;37(3):287–300.
3. Phillips KA. Suicidality in body dysmorphic disorder. Primary Psychiatry. 2007;2007(14):58–66.
4. Phillips KA, Albertini RS, Siniscalchi JM, Khan A, Robinson M. Effectiveness of pharmacotherapy for body dysmorphic disorder: a chart-review study. J Clin Psychiatry. 2001;62(9):721–7.

Suggested Readings

Mufaddel A, Osman OT, Almugaddam F, Jafferany M. A review of body dysmorphic disorder and its presentation in different clinical settings. Prim Care Companion CNS Disord. 2013;15(4).
Van Ameringen M, Patterson B, Simpson W. DSM-5 obsessive-compulsive and related disorders: clinical implications of new criteria. Depress Anxiety. 2014;31(6):487–93.

Chapter 3
Cassandra, the College Student

3.1 Case Presentation

Cassandra is a 19-year-old college sophomore in the US Midwest who presents in February to the student health center at the prompting of her resident advisor because of noticeable weight loss and concerns that she is restricting her food intake. Cassandra tells Ms. Dunning, the nurse practitioner doing her evaluation, that there is "no reason" for her to be here but that she was not given a choice. She explains that since returning to campus in the fall she has been trying to "get healthy," which she reports entails eating "lots of salad" and going to the gym every day. Cassandra elaborates that last year she gained "the freshman fifteen" during her first semester ("Actually, more like twenty. All-you-can-eat cereal —it's like they *want* us to blow up!!"); she was able to curtail her weight gain after that, but stayed at the higher weight for the rest of the year. Over the summer, she had tried to exercise more and watch what she was eating, but found it difficult because she would often be going out with her high school friends and that there were only "unhealthy options" from which to choose. She admits that her mother made a comment about her not fitting into her clothing

© Springer International Publishing Switzerland 2017
J. Gordon-Elliott, *Fundamentals of Diagnosing and Treating Eating Disorders*, DOI 10.1007/978-3-319-46065-9_3

the same way, which Cassandra found very upsetting. She describes her mother as "always skinny, always worried about her own weight... she totally has an eating disorder."

Upon returning to school in the fall, Cassandra found she was finally able cut calories, which she has been doing by eating only one bowl of cereal in the morning, having a banana and an apple for lunch most days, and eating a usual-sized dinner. This generally takes a good deal of restraint and leaves her hungry. There are occasions at night when she will "lose my willpower" because she still feels very hungry a few hours after dinner and she will eat more food before bed (e.g., going to the student union at 9 pm and sharing a large pizza with a friend and then having a medium cup of frozen yogurt). She describes feeling "disappointed" in herself the next morning after these instances, which had been happening approximately every two weeks; she will usually skip breakfast the next day, but otherwise not change her routine further.

She reports that she has lost about 25 lb between August and February. She admits that at her current weight of 145 lb (height 5′ 4″; body mass index [BMI] 24.9) she is "much happier" with the way she looks, liking that she can fit into a smaller size than she has been able to since freshman year of high school. She describes having many good friends and enjoying her classes, though she admits that her grades are a little below what they were last year, saying she sometimes has more difficulty concentrating on her studies if she has not eaten much during the day. She admits that she tried to purge twice but "couldn't make myself throw up—I hate throwing up!". She denies laxative use. She says she works out for about 45 min a day on the elliptical machine at the gym six days a week.

Upon further questioning, Cassandra elaborates that she had been an athletic child and adolescent, "a little chunkier" than most of the girls in her class and than her older sister, who has "always been super skinny like mom—you should be talking with the two of them, not me!". She reached menarche at age 12. She gained about 20 lb between ages 14 and 16, despite no further increase in her height. She describes having felt "pretty self-conscious" about her body in high school, with specific concerns about her "belly."

3.2 Diagnosis/Assessment

Preferred diagnosis: No diagnosis

Cassandra experiences some dissatisfaction with her appearance, and manipulation of her eating in response to that, but her symptoms most likely do not rise to the level of warranting a diagnosis.

Cassandra's story is, in many ways, quite typical. We hear in the story that this is a teenage girl who has had concerns about her body for many years, probably moderated by some degree of direct pressure (a mother who has, if not a diagnosable eating disorder, some impairment in her relationship with food and body image), and indirect influences, including media images and sociocultural standards of body ideals. Her self-estimation of being heavier than the average girl in her peer group growing up, and her weight gain during puberty, seem to have heightened her body dissatisfaction. Further weight gain in college triggered fairly substantial food restriction during this academic year, with resulting weight loss. At a calorie deficit (expending more calories than she is taking in), she feels hungry much of the time, with some subjective changes in her concentration. She periodically finds that it is hard to maintain the rigid calorie restriction, and she will eat more than usual, which she later regrets, making up for it with additional restriction the next day. More information should be sought from Cassandra to determine whether or not these eating episodes classify as binges (based on the quantity she eats and whether she experiences a sense of loss of control [see Chaps. 7 and 10 for further discussion about binge eating behavior]). To add to her calorie deficit, she engages in a moderate amount of exercise that would not be considered excessive, though arguably high given her overall calorie restriction. Her current BMI is at the upper limit of "normal weight." She is pleased with the changes in her appearance. She is still active socially and is endorsing no other psychiatric symptoms.

Cassandra's behavior has been excessive, perhaps—a fairly rigid, low-calorie diet, with a substantial weight loss over six months—but not substantially outside of the range of normal. In fact, studies indicate that some degree of preoccupation with body image concerns and dieting is more the norm than the exception in someone like Cassandra. Survey data show that upwards of 90 %

of college-aged women have dieted at some point to control their weight [5], and among all adolescents, nearly half of girls and a quarter of boys have used dieting or other disordered eating behaviors (including purging and related compensatory behaviors) [4]. Body dissatisfaction, which may be one of the primary moderators of the development of disordered eating and eating disorders, is extremely common in Western nations, with some survey data estimating that nearly 90 % of women in the USA are unhappy with their bodies; among youth, rates of body dissatisfaction are disturbingly high, with, for example, one study showing over 40 % of 1st–3rd grade girls expressing a desire to be "thinner" [1].

Cassandra's concerns about her body and her efforts to lose weight may—based purely on statistics—fall somewhere in the range of the "norm," but that is not reason enough to deem them "normal" and dismiss them. Body dissatisfaction is a significant risk factor for disordered eating and the development of full-syndrome eating disorders. In addition, it can contribute to low self-esteem, depression, anxiety, and impaired interpersonal relationships. Dieting, a benign enough word, can have substantial negative effects on an individual. When one is restricting calories, it is common to limit or remove certain food groups, leaving a diet that is deficient in certain macro- and micronutrients [see Chap. 12 for further information on general principles on balanced food intake and recommended dietary guidelines]. Losing weight rapidly may increase one's risk of regaining that weight quickly, with both medical and psychological sequelae. Significant fluctuations in weight over time may also have long-term effects on metabolic factors that determine calorie expenditure at rest, making it harder over time to lose weight. Food restriction also increases the chances of binge eating behavior [5], which carries risks, including the potential for weight gain and further development of disordered eating and compensatory behaviors.

Dieting may additionally have profound consequences on an individual's overall psychosocial functioning. Calorie restriction and preoccupation with food and body may lead to difficulties in concentration on other tasks, such as school or occupational pursuits. A person who is dieting may avoid social interactions where he or she might not be able to "follow" the diet. Irritability or

fatigue from an ongoing calorie deficit may impair one's relationships and performance at work. Moreover, dieting may be seen as a precursor to more pathological eating-related behavior. Among all people who diet, up to a third will progress to more extreme dieting, with a substantial number of those going on to develop full-syndrome eating disorders.

Because eating disorders can be very challenging to treat and take on a chronic course for many affected individuals, early identification and treatment are essential. Cassandra may not fulfill criteria for an eating disorder, and she may not fall that far from the "norm" in her peer group, but she is at risk for developing an eating disorder if her current symptoms persist or escalate. As college age is a prime time for the development of eating disorders (likely due to a combination of developmental and biological factors), there is high awareness about eating disorders on college campuses and among student advisors and counselors. Even though one would be correct in asserting that Cassandra does not have an eating disorder, it is appropriate that she was referred for further evaluation; if this student health evaluation identifies a problem and helps guide her toward healthier thoughts and behaviors, this early intervention could be lifesaving—*literally*.

Given how pervasive dieting behaviors and disordered eating symptoms are, it would be useful to have ways to identify which individuals are at the highest risk for progressing to pathologic eating behavior and full-syndrome eating disorders. We have some limited information to guide us. Risk factors for developing an eating disorder include female gender (this increased risk depends upon the specific disorder; for example, the ratio of females to males in anorexia nervosa and bulimia nervosa is approximately 10:1, while the ratio in binge eating disorder may be closer to 2:1 or 1:1); adolescence or early adulthood (though eating disorders exist at all ages and may persist as chronic disorders, it is most common for them to onset during this age range, and the prevalence in this group is highest); family history of eating disorders and personal history of other mental health disorders; dieting and body dissatisfaction; and competitive athletes [see Chap. 5 for further discussion about athletes and eating disorders] or those who engage in activities where appearance is a focus of significant attention (e.g., acting or modeling). Being overweight may also increase one's chances of engaging in more extreme dieting

behavior. It is worth noticing that rates of eating disorders have increased in parallel with an increase in rates of obesity and a culture with constant exposure and access to cheap, easy and boundless food options, such as fast food. Society and culture clearly influence the development of eating disorders, with these disorders being much more common in cultures that promote and value a thin ideal of beauty, and more common in individuals who have immigrated to Western nations compared those in their country of origin; moreover, prevalence of eating disorders has increased in tandem with the expansion of media images promoting and valuing thinness.

One can understand risk for developing eating disorders along a stress-diathesis model, where predisposing factors such as biological risk factors (e.g., family history, being overweight) and psychological and social influences (e.g., heavy exposure to images presenting unrealistic standards of thinness, and social pressures from friends or family to appear a certain way) are moderated by precipitants such as a period of high stress (for example, moving from one's family to college and facing independence and adulthood) and other triggers (such as losing a few pounds through a crash diet and receiving positive feedback from others), leading to the development of more pathological eating behavior and an eating disorder.

As prevalent as dieting, disordered eating behavior and body dissatisfaction are, it can be very challenging to determine which individuals are most at risk and most in need of intervention. Certain screening tools have been developed for use. The Questionnaire for Eating Disorder Diagnosis (Q-EDD) and the Eating Attitudes Test (EAT-26) are two self-administered screening tools with documented high sensitivity and specificity in clinical and non-clinical populations, though their use may be limited by time and patient engagement (50 and 26 questions in length, respectively). Shorter, clinician-administered screening tools—including the eating disorder screen for primary care (ESP) and the SCOFF—may be more feasible to use in primary care and general psychiatric practices, with variable sensitivity and specificity depending on setting and population (Table 3.1).

Table 3.1 Brief screening tools for eating disorders

ESP (eating disorder screen for primary care) [2]
• Are you satisfied with your eating patterns? (A "no" to this question was classified as an abnormal response)
• Do you ever eat in secret? (A "yes" to this and all other questions was classified as an abnormal response)
• Does your weight affect the way you feel about yourself?
• Have any members of your family suffered with an eating disorder?
• Do you currently suffer with or have you ever suffered in the past with an eating disorder?
SCOFF [3]
• Do you make yourself Sick because you feel uncomfortably full?
• Do you worry you have lost Control over how much you eat?
• Have you recently lost more than One stone (14 lbs or 7.7 kg) in a three-month period?
• Do you believe yourself to be Fat when others say you are thin?
• Would you say that Food dominates your life?

3.3 Differential Diagnosis

When evaluating Cassandra, Ms. Dunning would want to assess for the presence of a full-syndrome eating disorder. As Cassandra was not of low weight, she would not fulfill criteria for anorexia nervosa. Her episodes of eating more at night rarely involved eating enough to qualify as a binge (she was typically eating a somewhat larger than normal, but not excessive, portion); on occasion, she would eat a much larger amount and feel like she had no control to stop (consistent with a binge), but these episodes happened rarely. Based on this, the diagnoses of bulimia nervosa and binge eating disorder are not appropriate.

It could be argued that it would be appropriate to give her a diagnosis of *other specified feeding or eating disorder* (OSFED), which would describe subsyndromal symptoms and behaviors that are causing distress or impairment of functioning but not fully meeting the criteria of one of the DSM-5 feeding and eating disorder diagnoses. For example, if she were engaging in binge eating on a regular basis, causing significant impairment in an area of life functioning, but the binges were happening less frequently than once a week, she could be given the diagnosis of OSFED

(binge eating, with subsyndromal frequency). One diagnosis that has not yet been included as a separate diagnosis in the feeding and eating disorder chapter of DSM-5, but that has been described in the literature and is mentioned in the DSM, is *night eating syndrome* (NES). Individuals with NES will consume a large percent of their daily calories at night at least twice a week and will have associated distress or impairment associated with their symptoms. This diagnosis does not fit Cassandra's presentation on the basis of frequency, but would be something to consider and evaluate as part of the differential diagnosis.

Unspecified feeding or eating disorder is a preliminary diagnosis that would be given to an individual with eating disorder symptoms or behaviors that are causing distress or impairment but where there is not enough information at the time of assessment to further qualify the diagnosis with any specificity.

Spotlight on DSM-5

Several changes were made to the diagnoses that are currently included in the feeding and eating disorders chapter of DSM-5, including introducing three diagnoses that had previously been in an earlier section of the DSM focused on disorders of childhood; adjusting the criteria for anorexia nervosa and bulimia nervosa; and adding the diagnoses of other specified feeding or eating disorder (OSFED) and unspecified feeding or eating disorder (UFED). Experts had found that previous criteria for the major eating disorders were not inclusive enough to be applied to many individuals with significant eating disorder symptoms and behaviors that warranted clinical attention. Under DSM-IV, many of these individuals received a diagnosis of eating disorder not otherwise specified, which was actually found to be the most common eating disorder diagnosis given across populations. The resulting lumping together of a wide variety of eating pathology into one catchall group ("ED-NOS") was problematic, for both treatment and research purposes. Part of the intent of the OSFED classification is that it will allow presentations that seem consistent with one of the existing eating disorders, but that do not meet full criteria, to be given a

diagnosis with some specificity—e.g., "OSFED (symptoms consistent with bulimia nervosa, but binges occurring only once every other week)".

3.4 Outcome

Cassandra agreed to come back and see Ms. Dunning for a follow-up session, which Ms. Dunning facilitated by validating how hard it has been for Cassandra to "feel OK" about her body over the years and offering that together they could find ways for Cassandra to use the help of medical professionals to achieve an optimal weight in a healthy way. On her second visit, Cassandra spoke more about her lifelong sense of discomfort about her body size and shape ("I can remember worrying about fat when I was 5 years old, even though I wasn't fat!") and how she had attempted dieting at many points, but never for more than a day or two at a time. She recalled eating as a way to make her feel "better" when upset. She spoke at more length about being told to "watch my weight" by her mother, which generally only made her feel worse about herself. She was able to talk about how her body dissatisfaction stands in contrast to the appreciation she has always had with what her body was capable of as an athlete—she could point out how on the one hand she did not like her body, but on the other hand she took pride in the athletic achievements her body allowed her. Heavier in her junior and senior years of high school than she had been earlier on, she was often struck with a sense of "not looking the part" of the athlete that she was, but denies that she was ever encouraged by coaches or other athletes to focus on weight loss [see Chap. 5 for further discussion of athletes and eating disorders].

She admitted to Ms. Dunning that after losing the first 5–10 lb this year, she was getting a lot of positive feedback from her friends and that increased her desire to keep losing—"I can see how it could start to feel addictive." She also acknowledged that she has no sense of what her goal weight should be and no plan for how she will begin to normalize her eating in a way that would be sustainable over time. She expressed some fear that if she began

eating "more normally," she would "blow up and gain back all the weight and more."

Cassandra was referred to a nutritionist who worked with her to develop a balanced nutritional plan. She continued to see Ms. Dunning on a weekly basis to "talk about things." Over time, they spoke more about her relationship with her mother and worked on helping Cassandra take more satisfaction in her body. She joined an intramural soccer team, rediscovering how much joy she experienced engaging in sports. She made several good friends on the team, eating more of her meals with teammates over time and finding it easier to take pleasure in sharing mealtime with others, with less preoccupation with what or how much she was eating. Her weight remained stable for the rest of the academic year.

References

1. Collins ME. Body figure perceptions and preferences among pre-adolescent children. Int J Eat Disord. 1991;10(2):199–208.
2. Cotton MA, Ball C, Robinson P. Four simple questions can help screen for eating disorders. J Gen Intern Med. 2003;18:53–6.
3. Morgan JF, Reid F, Lacey H. The SCOFF questionnaire: assessment of a new screening tool for eating disorders. BMJ. 1999;319:1467–8.
4. Neumark-Sztainer D, Hannan PJ. Weight-related behaviors among adolescent girls and boys: results from a national survey. Arch Pediatr Adolesc Med. 2000;154(6):569–77.
5. Shisslak CM, Crago M, Estes LS. The Spectrum of eating disturbances. Int J Eat Disord. 1995;18(3):209–19.

Suggested Readings

Boutelle K, Neumark-Sztainer D, Story M, Resnick M. Weight control behaviors among obese, overweight, and nonoverweight adolescents. J Pediatr Psychol. 2002;27:531–40.
Crow S, Eisenberg ME, Story M, Neumark-Sztainer D. Suicidal behavior in adolescents: relationship to weight status, weight control behaviors, and body dissatisfaction. Int J Eat Disord. 2008;41(1):82–7.
Hogan MJ, Strasburger VC. Body image, eating disorders, and the media. Adolesc Med State Art Rev. 2008;19(3):521–46, x–xi.

http://www.researchgate.net/profile/Shelly_Grabe/publication/6963208_Ethni
    city_and_body_dissatisfaction_among_women_in_the_United_States_a_
    meta-analysis/links/54302ca40cf277d58e966479.pdf.
Neumark-Sztainer D, Bauer KW, Friend S, Hannan PJ, Story M, Berge JM.
    Family weight talk and dieting: how much do they matter for body
    dissatisfaction and disordered eating behaviors in adolescent girls? J
    Adolesc Health. 2010;47(3):270–6.
The 1997 Body Image Survey Results. Psychology Today. Jan–Feb, 1997.

Chapter 4
Danny, the Picky Eater

4.1 Case Presentation

Danny is a 7-year-old boy brought in to see his pediatrician, Dr. Ellis, by his parents because of "picky eating." Danny's parents explain that Danny has "never been a great eater," always requiring more time to complete his feeding or meals than his two older brothers, and being generally averse to the introduction of new food items, but for the past six months, he has become markedly more challenging to feed, refusing most foods other than white bread and undressed pasta. They report that when presented with other foods, such as vegetables, he will push them off his plate. In the cases where the family is able to get him to eat other items, he will make an expression of distress or tell them that it tastes like broccoli (he has taken to calling all foods of any color, including fruits, vegetables, and even many meats, "broccoli"). Mealtime at the dinner table will often result in his crying, so his parents have begun allowing him to eat at a small table in the corner of the room while the rest of the family eats at the main table. He still drinks water, milk, and apple juice. He will eat jelly on his bread when at school (but not at home).

Danny has been appearing more quiet to his parents, often preferring to play alone rather than with his older brother. His

© Springer International Publishing Switzerland 2017
J. Gordon-Elliott, *Fundamentals of Diagnosing and Treating Eating Disorders*, DOI 10.1007/978-3-319-46065-9_4

father comments that Danny has also been demanding to wear the same sweater day after day, and they have on occasion seen him taking it on and off repeatedly while he is by himself. He has no other physical symptoms, such as vomiting. His parents do note that a couple of weeks before they first noticed these symptoms, Danny had had a sore throat, which resolved over the course of a few days. His parents were hoping that this was "just a phase" but have become increasingly concerned, especially as they are now getting input from the school that he is crying when other children have birthdays and bring in cupcakes for the class (which he refuses to eat). He also has been complaining of "tummy aches" when over at friends' houses for playdates, often prompting him to be brought home early.

Dr. Ellis' examination demonstrates that Danny is a thin, young boy, though energetic and otherwise appearing well. His weight has not increased since his last checkup 5 months prior. His physical examination is otherwise unrevealing. He engages as he typically does with Dr. Ellis—reserved and sometimes noted to be clinging to his mother, but answering questions when asked. He communicates clearly and appears to have an age-appropriate vocabulary. Dr. Ellis is considering a gastroenterology consultation to assess for mechanical issues preventing Danny from eating normally, as well as for any allergies or food intolerance that might be causing him to avoid certain items.

4.2 Diagnosis/Assessment

Preferred diagnosis: Avoidant Restrictive Food Intake Disorder (ARFID).

The most suitable diagnosis in this case is ARFID, a new diagnosis to DSM-5 (a variant under the name feeding disorder of infancy and childhood existed in DSM-IV [see Text box: *Spotlight on DSM-5: ARFID*]). ARFID can be diagnosed in children and adults, and it describes a pattern of food avoidance in the absence of body image issues or a wish to lose weight [see Text Box: ARFID: DSM-5 Diagnostic Criteria].

A newly defined diagnosis, little is yet known about the prevalence of ARFID in the general population. Small studies have

documented a prevalence of approximately 15 % among children and adolescents presenting to specialized eating disorder treatment programs [2].

It is thought that ARFID typically has an onset in childhood and adolescence, though it can begin later in life. Individuals with ARFID may have a history of always being "picky eaters," or the onset of food avoidance behavior may present more abruptly. The eating behavior itself may vary. For some individuals, the food avoidance may follow an eating-related event, such as choking on a specific food item (in which case, the disorder begins more as a typical phobia); for others, there may appear to be more of a focus on specific elements of the food that are experienced with disgust or anxiety, such as textural or taste components. For some, the avoidance may seem more arbitrary, such as individuals who refuse all food of a certain color, for example.

Little is known about the underlying biological, psychological, or social determinants of ARFID; at this point, the diagnosis is largely defined phenomenologically.

For a child or adult who is experiencing specific food aversions, the evaluation should first focus on an appropriate medical work-up. For example, if the individual is describing symptoms, or exhibiting signs, of choking or even vomiting, upper gastroenterological disorders of the esophagus or stomach may need to be ruled out. As another example, avoidance of specific food items should raise the possibility of allergic or intolerance issues. In the setting of new signs and symptoms, it would be reasonable to start with a thorough evaluation by a general medical practitioner, with judicious use of invasive testing and interventions where indicated.

In addition to any pertinent medical evaluation, the individual should undergo a full psychiatric assessment, evaluating for the presence of a variety of psychiatric disorders (see *Differential Diagnosis*, below). Once the diagnosis of ARFID has been determined, a treatment plan should be outlined, including nutritional evaluation and counseling, and engagement in behavioral treatment to help modify abnormal eating behaviors that are preventing adequate nutritional intake. As many of those with this disorder are still children and adolescents, engaging the family in the treatment is often essential. It is not uncommon for family members to develop their own emotional and behavioral responses to the patient's symptoms—from increased anxiety, to harsh or critical

reactions, to avoidance—all of which can contribute to the patient's food avoidance and abnormal eating. Careful monitoring of weight, with specific goals for restoration of a healthy weight and related physical parameters, as well as collaboration between mental health and medical providers, are important elements of the treatment of patients with ARFID.

Spotlight on DSM-5: ARFID

One of the major organizational and conceptual changes from DSM-IV-TR to DSM-5 was the removal of the splitting of diagnoses into two sections based on typical age of onset. In DSM-IV, the book opened with a chapter containing the "Disorders Usually First Diagnosed in Infancy, Childhood, and Adolescence," followed by chapters reviewing the diagnoses that typically onset during adulthood. This first section included such disorders as the developmental and intellectual disorders and attention deficit hyperactivity disorder, as well as a few disorders of feeding and eating, including pica, rumination syndrome, and feeding disorder of infancy and childhood. This last diagnosis described individuals who developed a pattern of food avoidance before age six, without a medical cause or a lack of access to food to account for the symptoms, and evidence of inadequate nutritional intake. This categorical separation of disorders into childhood and adult disorders was eliminated in DSM-5, with the rationale that there can be substantial overlap (with some disorders more "typical" of adult onset beginning in childhood and vice versa), and because this arbitrary separation was not thought to have a clear evidence base or clinical meaning. In DSM-5, these DSM-IV childhood feeding and eating disorders were combined with the eating disorders found later in the book and reorganized into the chapter, "Feeding and Eating Disorders."

Feeding disorder of infancy and childhood was adapted into ARFID with the elimination of the age of onset cut-off, and more flexibility included in terms of the presence of a medical disorder. With ARFID, the symptoms may therefore onset at any age, and there can be a medical issue that might contribute to symptoms, but—in such a case—the symptoms

are considered to be out of proportion of what would be expected from that medical disorder. These changes allow more flexibility in how this diagnosis is used, potentially capturing more cases which previously would have been given a diagnosis of ED-NOS, or otherwise missed.

Avoidant Restrictive Food Intake Disorder: DSM-5 Diagnostic Criteria

A. An eating or feeding disturbance as manifested by persistent failure to meet appropriate nutritional and/or energy needs associated with one (or more) of the following:

  1. Significant weight loss (or failure to achieve expected weight gain or faltering growth in children).
  2. Significant nutritional deficiency.
  3. Dependence on enteral feeding or oral nutritional supplements.
  4. Marked interference with psychosocial functioning.

B. The disturbance is not better explained by a lack of available food or by an associated culturally sanctioned practice.

C. The eating disturbance does not occur exclusively during the course of anorexia nervosa or bulimia nervosa, and there is no evidence of a disturbance in the way in which one's body weight or shape is experienced.

D. The eating disturbance is not attributable to a concurrent medical condition (when a medical condition is present, the severity of the eating disturbance exceeds what would be expected) or not better explained by another mental disturbance.

4.3 Differential Diagnosis

The differential diagnosis for ARFID is broad, including a range of psychiatric and medical conditions, as well as variants of normal behavior.

Patients with suspected ARFID should be screened for other eating disorders, most importantly anorexia nervosa (AN) because of substantial overlap between these disorders in terms of their presentations and clinical features [See Text Box: Focus on Differential Diagnosis for additional discussion]. Pica and rumination disorder, both eating disorders that commonly present in childhood, may result in poor calorie intake and weight loss or lack of appropriate weight gain [see Chap. 13 for further discussion]. Additional disorders related to food and eating that currently would fall under the categories of unspecified feeding or eating disorder or other specified feeding or eating disorder, such as preoccupation with eating in a "healthy" way, or avoidance of certain foods due to self-perceived "allergies" or "intolerances," should be considered [for additional discussion of these types of presentations, see Chaps. 14, 15, and 16].

Anxiety disorders that may impact a person's eating patterns or comfort with eating may coexist or contribute to the eating symptoms. In social anxiety disorder, an individual may be particularly concerned about how he or she would be perceived while eating, or eating certain foods, and may therefore change eating behavior to minimize this anxiety. If the food refusal only involves one particular type of food for which the patient has an explicit phobia (e.g., a fear of choking on one identified food item), then a diagnosis of specific phobia might be considered; however, if there are other features fulfilling the criteria of a diagnosis of ARFID, the latter would be the more appropriate diagnosis as it would determine the focus of clinical attention and treatment. Obsessive compulsive disorder might involve specific concerns about food items, or rituals involved in eating, that prevent adequate nutritional intake. Individuals with autism spectrum disorders may have ritualized ways of eating, hypersensitivity to certain sensory aspects of food such as taste or texture, or behavioral disturbances that interfere with eating. Lastly, various medical issues that prevent or influence eating behaviors, such as gastrointestinal disorders or allergic conditions, can present with symptoms consistent with ARFID; an effort should be made to determine whether the eating symptoms can be fully attributed to the medical disorder or, rather, are considered out of proportion to what would be expected.

Focus on Differential Diagnosis

What distinguishes ARFID from AN is the focus on weight and body image (see Chap. 1 for further discussion of AN). Patients with ARFID may present and behave very similarly to those with AN. A patient with ARFID may be underweight and may have experienced weight loss or (in the case of a developing child or adolescent) may have not met expected gains in weight; patients with both diagnoses may avoid certain foods and become distressed when anticipating or being compelled to ingest those foods; and they both may behave in ways that prevent maintenance of a healthy weight or nutritional state. For example, a teenager who is persistently refusing to eat adequate amounts of food, and is denying a wish to be thin but nonetheless is maintaining a low body weight due to food refusal, could theoretically receive a diagnosis of ARFID or AN. The central difference between the two, however, is that the patient with AN is preoccupied with body size and maintenance of a low weight, while the focus in ARFID is the avoidance of certain food or food groups, without the additional goal of achieving or maintaining a very low weight. This distinction might be challenging to determine in some individuals. If the diagnosis of AN is strongly suspected, this should most likely be the initial emphasis of clinical attention, and if the eating disturbance has only occurred during the course of active AN symptoms, then a diagnosis of ARFID cannot be made.

Some differences may differentiate these two disorders. In a study of children and adolescents presenting to an eating disorders program, compared to individuals with AN, youngsters with ARFID were more likely to be male, younger, and more likely to have a medical condition or physical symptoms [1].

For both diagnoses, the treatment, at least initially, will be primarily focused on behavioral modification to engage the patient in developing more normal and sustainable eating habits. Supervised refeeding in inpatient or outpatient settings may be required for those who are very underweight or who have medical complications from being low weight.

In AN, further psychotherapeutic focus may be on the underlying beliefs and emotions related to body image, while in ARFID there may be additional exploration of specific fears or aversions to particular food items.

4.4   Outcome

The diagnosis of ARFID is an important one to make, as—without identification the correct diagnosis—individuals with this condition may either be subject to unnecessary medical testing and iatrogenic harm, or go unrecognized and not receive appropriate treatment for the restoration of emotional and physical health. Without treatment, these individuals may progress to having substantial medical sequelae of poor nutrition. In addition, they may go on to develop other eating disorders, such as AN. As this clinical entity, as currently defined, is new, there are limited data at this time about natural history and outcome with adequate treatment. More longitudinal assessment and research of this disorder are needed to expand the evidence base and to offer guidance on best practices for individuals with ARFID.

In the case of Danny, after a basic evaluation by his pediatrician that did not identify any major medical issues contributing to his food refusal, Danny and his parents began family-based behavioral treatment. After a brief psychoeducation, his parents were trained to use rewards in response to healthy eating habits and specific guidelines for promoting effective nutritional intake by limiting distractions at mealtimes, giving time limits for eating, and not allowing for food item substitutions or other food-related negotiations. His parents were able to talk with the therapist about their own emotional responses to Danny's food refusal, and to slowly identify ways in which their anxiety about his symptoms was manifesting at mealtimes and any time food was discussed or considered; with additional counseling, they were able to process these feelings more effectively and not have them influence their interactions with Danny, helping them to gain more of a sense of control over the situation. Danny gradually began to gain weight at

a rate more appropriate for his age, and to catch up to a more healthy growth curve. He started eating a wider range of foods. His emotional disturbances at school lessened, and his interactions with other children improved. As the eating symptoms subsided, it became more clear that there were anxiety symptoms independent of the eating disorder, consistent with a diagnosis of generalized anxiety disorder, and he began receiving therapy for his anxiety disorder with good response.

References

1. Fisher MM, Rosen DS, Ornstein RM, Mammel KA, Katzman DK, Rome ES, Callahan ST, Malizio J, Kearney S, Walsh BT. Characteristics of avoidant/restrictive food intake disorder in children and adolescents: a "new disorder" in DSM-5. J Adolesc Health. 2014;55(1):49–52.
2. Ornstein RM, Rosen DS, Mammel KA, Callahan ST, Forman S, Jay MS, Fisher M, Rome E, Walsh BT. Distribution of eating disorders in children and adolescents using the proposed DSM-5 criteria for feeding and eating disorders. J Adolesc Health. 2013;53:303–5.

Suggested Readings

Bryant-Waugh R. Feeding and eating disorder in children. Curr Opin Psychiatry. 2013;26:537–42.
Norris ML, Katzman DK. Change is never easy, but it is possible: reflections on avoidant/restrictive food intake disorder two years after its introduction in the DSM-5. J Adolesc Health. 2015;57:8–9.

Chapter 5
Eric, the Hopeful Olympian

5.1 Case Presentation

Eric is a 24-year-old man seeing his primary care doctor,
Dr. Frank, for evaluation of "fatigue." During his initial evaluation,
Eric—who is currently a full-time runner with hopes of qualifying
for the 10-km competition in the next Olympic Games—explains
that he has been sleeping poorly for the past 6–9 months, with
difficulty falling asleep, early morning awakening, and feeling tired
and "worn down all the time." Eric, a successful collegiate runner,
chose to pursue an elite running career after graduating college. He
continued working with his college coach and was sharing a house
with runner friends, while working part-time at a local running
store. After some early disappointing races, Eric decided that he
might perform better if he lost 5 lb to achieve the weight he had
raced at in his junior year, which had been his most successful
season. It was easy to lose this weight with a small reduction in
calorie intake and an increase in his weekly mileage. Over the next
12 months, still unable to improve his performance to the level he
thought was within his capacity, Eric became more focused on his
diet and weight, gradually reducing his intake further and forgoing
speed workouts and group runs with his teammates for long runs
on his own to try to increase his mileage further. He felt his job at

© Springer International Publishing Switzerland 2017   43
J. Gordon-Elliott, *Fundamentals of Diagnosing and Treating
Eating Disorders*, DOI 10.1007/978-3-319-46065-9_5

the running store was getting in the way of his running, and quit the job. He began considering switching to a new coach or relocating. He was spending less time with his housemates and more time in his bedroom, reading and stretching. He found himself worrying about his future and what would come of him if he did not achieve his professional running goals.

By the time he saw Dr. Frank, 18 months after graduation from college, he was 20 lb below his senior-year weight, with a BMI of 17.5. He felt cold all the time, tired and unfocused. He described a very restricted diet, in terms of range of food items and overall calories. He admitted that "on occasion" he got so hungry that he would eat much larger amounts in a short period of time; he would then reduce his intake the next day and add a few more miles to his run. He reported a low mood. He had difficulty falling and staying asleep, feeling constantly "on edge." He hoped Dr. Frank could offer a medication to help him sleep better, so he might be able to train at a higher level.

5.2   Diagnosis/Assessment

Preferred diagnosis: The most appropriate diagnosis for Eric is anorexia nervosa (AN) [for more discussion of AN, see Chap. 1]. Eric has been restricting his calories with increasing preoccupation about maintaining a very low weight and fear about gaining weight. In addition, he has become more focused on his weight as a measure of his self-worth and identity, such that his weight on any given day has a substantial impact on how he feels about himself. His drive for thinness has surpassed its initial purpose; what developed in attempt to enhance performance has now seemed to have led to a decline in performance and impairment in several areas of functioning.

For many reasons, the diagnosis of AN might be missed or discounted in Eric's case—most relevant here, Eric is male and an athlete. Eating disorders in general, and AN specifically, are significantly more prevalent in females, with a reported 10:1 female predominance in AN. This statistic, however, should highlight that AN is in fact not an exclusively female disorder, and clinicians should be mindful of the small but significant population of males with AN. Moreover, because the typical AN patient is female, it is

important to note that a boy or man with AN may have clinical features that differ somewhat from the classic perception of the disorder. Whereas a female patient, due to various factors including pervasive cultural norms and social acceptability, might be more likely to explicitly link her maintenance of low weight to her body image, a male patient might not report body image as a motivating factor. He might, for example, be more likely to attribute his low weight and refusal to gain weight to an athletic performance goal. This will be particularly common in men who participate in sports that involve vertical motion where being at a very lean weight enhances performance, such as middle- and long-distance running, as well as those sports that involve weight classes, such as wrestling, where there is a potential advantage to being in the upper range of a weight class below one's natural body type.

Males with eating disorders may be more likely than women to have a history of being overweight before the development of the eating disorder and to have more general psychiatric comorbidity; males with eating disorders may be diagnosed later in the course of illness than females, perhaps in part due to assumptions that eating disorders are largely exclusive to girls and women. Homosexual males appear to be at higher risk for developing eating disorders than heterosexual males.

As the case of Eric demonstrates, the diagnosis of an eating disorder in competitive athletes, male and female, may be more challenging to make and at risk of being missed. Elite and otherwise competitive athletes will manipulate their food intake and exercise to optimize their performance. As mentioned previously, some athletic endeavors, such as those requiring vertical motion like running and dancing, are typically better performed the leaner an athlete is (though excessive leanness to the detriment of essential stores of fat mass will ultimately begin to hamper performance). Other sports involve weight classes, where an athlete may actively manipulate his or her weight to be at the upper limit of a weight class at the time of the precompetition weigh-in. Weight control may include cutting calories, or limiting specific macronutrients (such as carbohydrates, in the case where water weight needs to be kept at a minimum—for example, before a wrestling match weigh-in). Athletes may add in extra calorie-burning exercise in order to expend more energy and bring weight down. Some additional compensatory behaviors, including

wearing extra clothing in order to lose more fluid in sweat as a temporary measure before a weigh-in, are not uncommon practice. Among certain groups, behaviors that might be considered frankly disordered in the general population may be almost normative, with extreme dieting or purging of food subtly or not so subtly encouraged by teammates or even a coach.

In some sports, there may be an aesthetic ideal that the athletes will strive for as it is so integrally related to the sport, itself. For example, achievement in long-distance running is seen typically in very lean individuals. Runners with varying body types may make efforts to emulate that lean archetype—as a concrete demonstration that they "fit in" and can similarly be top performers. This may occur even in athletes who, for reasons to do with their individual physiologies, would perform better with a less lean physique. In ballet or ice-skating, as other examples, there may be an idealized body type that is considered more appealing, based on the cultural standards within the sport; these ideals may not just be more "beautiful to the eye" but may actually be unconsciously experienced by the judge or audience member to be associated with a higher level of performance (e.g., a certain body type for a female skater, if more bulky or overtly muscular, may influence the judges' evaluations on an implicit level that the judges would not recognize they are doing).

When would a diagnosis of an eating disorder be made in athletes in such cases? This will depend upon the individual and will require a careful evaluation of the athlete's relationship to his or her body and food. The signs may be subtle—the athlete started reducing calories based on the recommendations of the coach and nutritionist, but over time, the athlete begins to demonstrate more anxiety around eating, more preoccupation with his or her weight, and gradual reduction of activities that might threaten his or her eating and weight maintenance (e.g., social gatherings). The athlete may develop a disproportionate amount of self-esteem related to the number on the scale or the body fat measure, rather than on athletic performance, itself. The athlete may continue to engage in calorie reduction or extra calorie expenditure even in the face of worsening results, such as slipping race times. Additional indications that behavior which initially began for performance enhancement has become pathological could include the inability to "relax" one's rules and restrictions around calorie intake and expenditure during the "off-season" or on rest days.

In general, it might be recommended that if there is a concern that an individual's behaviors related to food and exercise are putting him or her at risk medically, or causing undue psychological distress (excessive preoccupation, impairment of social or occupational functioning, etc.), it would be reasonable to have a low threshold for considering an eating disorder and to address it as such. A complicating factor will be that the individual will likely have numerous explanations for his or her behavior, all to do with performance enhancement or the culture of the sport (often frankly denying a desire for thinness due to body image purposes, per se) and may be highly resistant to any intervention. The athlete may experience the mental health provider who is attempting to offer help as trying to obstruct performance and athletic development. These individuals, therefore, may be best approached by others in the sport—e.g., a trusted coach or the team physician, psychologist, and nutritionist. Even in such cases, however—just as is found in the management of feeding and eating disorders, in general—it can be tremendously challenging to gain the trust of a patient struggling with an eating disorder and to generate motivation to change behavior.

Regardless of the confounding factors, Eric's case illustrates quite characteristically the process that so commonly results in the development of AN. An initial focus on losing a few pounds, perhaps for aesthetic reasons or—as for Eric—athletic performance, leads to an increased focus on weight and calorie intake and expenditure. Reinforcement for early weight loss (e.g., a sense of accomplishment or positive feedback from others) may result, in an individual with certain biological and psychological vulnerabilities, in the "catching on" of weight loss, such that the individual is soon engaged in a constant pursuit of lowering his weight, with increasing efforts required to accomplish this and progressive focus on it, gradually encroaching upon multiple areas of functioning and preoccupying his existence.

The evaluation should include a careful review of Eric's stated motivations for his eating and exercise behaviors, with a special attention to indications that his weight and body are unduly influencing his sense of self-esteem and identity, or impacting his functioning in negative ways. He should be evaluated for other compensatory behaviors that he may be engaging in, such as vomiting or laxative use. He should be screened for mood symptoms and anxiety symptoms that could indicate other psychiatric

conditions that warrant clinical attention. When assessing eating disorder symptoms in athletes, it is important to tease out whether the athlete's emphasis is on pursuit of thinness (as in the case of Eric) or the pursuit of muscularity; if the latter is true, a diagnosis of body dysmorphic disorder, muscle dysmorphia subtype, might be the more appropriate diagnosis [see Chap. 2 for further discussion]. The medical evaluation should incorporate physiological parameters that may be affected by calorie and micro- and macronutrient deficiencies, including assessing for anemia, vitamin and mineral deficiencies, and osteopenia/osteoporosis.

5.3 Differential Diagnosis

The differential diagnosis for anorexia nervosa in Eric's case should include other eating disorders, including bulimia nervosa, and the degree and type of compensatory behaviors should be noted. In Eric's case, his intermittent eating of large amounts of food and his use of excessive energy expenditure to reverse calorie intake could fit criteria for bulimia nervosa. However, because his weight is maintained at a significantly low weight, it would be more appropriate to consider this AN, with the possibility of qualifying as the "binge-eating/purging" subtype.

Also in the differential diagnosis is an anxiety disorder or a depressive disorder. Generalized anxiety disorder and major depressive disorder, for example, could be further screened for and diagnosed if appropriate. If present, these would not exclude the diagnosis of AN or another eating disorder. Medical conditions that could be contributing to some of the physical and cognitive/ emotional symptoms should also be considered (and may in some cases be a result of the athlete's restricted diet), including disorders of the thyroid, anemia, or vitamin or mineral deficiencies.

Lastly, an individual like Eric might be considered to not have an eating disorder—rather, that his eating and weight management are a function of his athletic pursuits. However, in Eric's case, attributing his behavior to normal athletic training would miss the opportunity to intervene and help him. His eating and exercise behaviors have surpassed those standards that most athletes would consider normal, and his performance is suffering. His weight is having undue impact on his sense of his identity. His behaviors are

substantially impacting his overall functioning. At this point, to not diagnose an eating disorder and offer help would be missing an important clinical problem and could lead to ongoing symptoms and further morbidity and functional decline.

Spotlight on Eating Disorders in Competitive Athletes
Athletes who participate in competitive sports and elite athletic activities are at higher risk for developing eating disorders and disordered eating than the general population. Female athletes are perhaps particularly at risk with some studies suggesting that up to one-third of competitive high school athletes, and nearly one half of collegiate athletes, have a diagnosis of an eating disorder, while more than one half of high school and college female athletes have some degree of subclinical eating disorders characterized by an unhealthy relationship to calorie intake and expenditure. Though these numbers vary according to the study and may be sport-specific, what is clear is that competitive athletes face higher-than-average risk of developing an eating disorder, with all the medical and mental health consequences that these bring. The "female athlete triad" is the combination of disordered eating, loss of menses, and osteoporosis, with short- and long-term ramifications. Athletic organizations, including the NCAA, have been increasingly aware of the prevalence of eating disorders in athletes, and many have formal position statements on the subject, including recommendations for screening. Several screening tools have been developed for detecting eating disorders and subclinical disordered eating in athletes, including the Survey of Eating Disorders among Athletes (SEDA), the Female Athlete Screening Tool (FAST), and the Athlete Milieu Direct Questionnaire (AMDQ) [1].

5.4 Outcome

Eric described increasing anxiety about his body and his food, and expanding preoccupation on how many calories he was burning and eating. He described feeling unable to fit in other activities which used

to bring him pleasure, including spending time with friends and family. With time, he was able to admit that his eating and exercise requirements were feeling like overwhelming burdens to him, and yet he felt unable to change the cycle out of a vague fear that everything in his life might "come crashing down." Dr. Frank engaged a nutritionist colleague who worked primarily with elite athletes to see Eric; in their work together, Eric was able to see how his manipulation of food and exercise was going beyond the limits of what other top athletes were doing. Eric was able to gradually accept Dr. Frank's impression that his eating and exercise had gone past the threshold of pursuit of athletic performance and had become a problem and accepted a referral to a therapist. With time and engagement with the nutritionist and his coach, Eric was able to gradually increase his food intake and reduce his exercise. Cautiously, he continued to compete, with substantial attention to not allowing him to "cross that line" again. His performance improved and he began to enjoy the training and competing again. He did not qualify for the Olympic trials the next time they were offered and he was not placing well in the top meets; after much deliberation and counsel, Eric chose to stop pursuing a career running as an elite athlete. He began coaching runners and continued to run competitively, but not professionally, and to do so with great pleasure.

Reference

1. Knapp J, Aerni G, Anderson J. Eating disorders in female athletes: use of screening tools. Curr Sports Med Rep. 2014;13(4):214–8.

Suggested Readings

Arcelus J, Witcomb GL, Mitchell A. Prevalence of eating disorders among dancers: a systemic review and meta-analysis. Eur Eat Disorders Rev. 2014;22:92–101.

Raevuori A, Keski-Rahkonen A, Hoek HW. A review of eating disorders in males. Curr Opin Psychiatry. 2014;27(6):426–30.

Sundgot-Borgen J, Torstveit MK. Prevalence of eating disorders in elite athletes is higher than in the general population. Clin J Sport Med. 2004;14 (1):25–32.

Chapter 6
Francine's Insulin Issues

6.1 Case Presentation

Francine is a 16-year-old girl with type 1 diabetes diagnosed at age 11, referred by her endocrinologist, Dr. Ward, to Dr. Green, a psychiatrist, for evaluation of "non-compliance". Dr. Ward explains that Francine had always been "a very good girl," but over the past several months, her glycemic control has been poor, and she has been noted to be more irritable during her checkups, dismissing his concerns, snapping at her parents, and taking out her phone to check her social media updates. She has also lost 7 lb over 5 months (current height 5′6″, weight 130 lb, BMI 21). Dr. Ward suspects that she has been taking her insulin erratically, leading to elevated blood sugars and weight loss.

On Dr. Green's evaluation, Francine reports that she uses her insulin "like I'm supposed to" and attributes her weight loss to "being busy." Her parents tell Dr. Green that Francine has been avoiding eating with them at dinnertime, asking to eat her meals alone in her room, where she is "always on the computer or her phone." Since her diagnosis, they have helped to manage her insulin, but she has been refusing their involvement recently. They express concern about her weight loss and worry she may have an eating disorder. A rhythmic gymnast from age 9 to 13, Francine

© Springer International Publishing Switzerland 2017
J. Gordon-Elliott, *Fundamentals of Diagnosing and Treating
Eating Disorders*, DOI 10.1007/978-3-319-46065-9_6

had always been "petite", but began gaining weight around the
time she began taking insulin. Her parents report that for the past 3
years, she has occasionally spoken about feeling "fat", and that
beginning a year ago, she has been frequently crying when getting
ready for school (shouting sometimes at her mother, "my clothes
don't fit!"), and becoming more argumentative when shopping for
new clothes. Her mother reports that she once walked into
Francine's room and saw on the computer screen an image of an
emaciated-appearing teenage girl looking at herself in the mirror,
but Francine quickly closed the image and refused to explain what
she was viewing. During the session, Dr. Green says to Francine
that sometimes teens may skip insulin doses in order to lose
weight—asking, "have you ever tried that?" Francine's response is
an angry, "that sounds crazy."

6.2   Diagnosis/Assessment

Preferred diagnosis: other specified feeding or eating disorder
(normal weight; insulin overuse for weight loss).

Francine exemplifies the kind of patient that can be commonly
seen in primary care and specialty medical practice, as well as
general psychiatric practice—a patient who seems to have substantial concerns about body image and weight, and who is most
likely manipulating her eating and calorie balance (in her case,
through insulin omission), but who may not cleanly fit into a
specific feeding or eating disorder. This presentation is common
enough to have been colloquially labeled "diabulimia".

At the time that Francine's endocrinologist referred her to see
Dr. Green, Francine was not underweight and—at least during this
initial evaluation—was denying engaging in excessive means to
lose weight; she therefore would not (at least while she still
maintains a normal weight) fulfill criteria for anorexia nervosa
(AN; see Chap. 1 for more discussion of this diagnosis). She was
also denying binge-eating episodes and, as such, was not fitting a
diagnosis of bulimia nervosa (BN; see Chap. 7 for more discussion
of this diagnosis). On the other hand, her parents were sensing

clues that raised their suspicion for an eating disorder, including Francine's increased preoccupation with her body shape and weight. With further evaluation by Dr. Green over a few sessions, it becomes clear that Francine is taking measures to lose weight, including both calorie restriction and insulin omission, and she is doing this in the setting of body dissatisfaction. Francine has an eating disorder, and—despite its not fitting neatly into one of the major feeding or eating disorder diagnoses—it is important to identify the condition and address it; left untreated, this pattern of problematic eating-related behavior and distorted ideas about body image may progress, resulting in substantial psychiatric and medical morbidity.

Dr. Green assigns the diagnosis of other specified feeding or eating Disorder (normal weight; insulin overuse for weight loss). OSFED [see Text box: OSFED: DSM-5 Diagnostic Criteria], a diagnosis new to the DSM-5 [see Text box: Spotlight on DSM-5: OSFED], should be used when there are relevant symptoms of an eating disorder considered worthy of clinical attention, where the symptoms do not fit into one of the specified diagnoses but the nature of the eating disorder can be described in specific terms. In Francine's case, she remains within normal weight and is misusing insulin and calorie restriction for weight loss.

OSFED: DSM-5 Diagnostic Criteria

This diagnosis should be applied to presentations consistent with a feeding or eating disorder, causing clinically significant distress or impairment, but not meeting full criteria for one of the designated disorders. The diagnosis is listed as OSFED, followed by specific descriptors.

Some examples might include (but are not limited to) the following:

1. Aytpical anorexia nervosa: All of the criteria for anorexia nervosa are met except that, despite significant weight loss, the individual's weight is within or above the normal range.

2. Bulimia nervosa (of low frequency and/or limited duration): All of the criteria for bulimia nervosa are met, except that that binge eating and inappropriate compensatory behaviors occur, on average, less than once a week and/or for less than 3 months
3. Binge eating disorder (of low frequency and/or limited duration)
4. Purging disorder
5. Night eating syndrome

Spotlight on DSM-5: OSFED

New to DSM-5, other specified feeding or eating disorder (OSFED) was intended to address one of the limitations of the eating disorder classifications in DSM-IV—namely, that at least half of the individuals with clinically significant eating disorders were receiving a too broad diagnosis of eating disorder not otherwise specified (EDNOS). OSFED allows the clinician to identify an eating disorder that does not fulfill criteria for one of the existing diagnoses (e.g., due to not meeting the required frequency threshold of symptoms, or because of atypical features), while stating in parentheses the nature of the eating disorder. The development of the "Other Specified" diagnosis, included in most diagnostic categories of the DSM-5, encourages more diagnostic precision, with implications on clinical care and research.

Unspecified feeding or eating disorder should be used in the case of a presentation that does not meet the criteria for one of the other disorders, but for which not enough information is yet known to qualify or describe the nature of the disorder (for example, after a single evaluation in an Emergency Room setting).

6.2.1   Eating Disorders and Chronic Medical Illness

Chronic illness in childhood and adolescence can impact psychosocial development in a variety of ways, with repercussions on physical and mental health outcomes. Some youngsters may become fastidious about managing their illness, attempting to control the aspects of their behavior and environment that influence the disease; though adaptive in moderation, this response can lead to anxiety and other mental health issues when taken to more of an extreme. Other youngsters may reject the excessive control that has been required of them over the years to manage the illness, becoming non-adherent with medical care and engaging in maladaptive health behaviors, such as poor diet or substance use issues.

Eating disorders, including AN, BN, and binge eating disorder (BED), have been found to be more prevalent among patients with type 1 and type 2 diabetes. Several factors related to living with diabetes may put adolescents and young adults with the disease at higher risk for developing an eating disorder. For individuals with type 1 (and in some cases, type 2) diabetes, weight loss occurs prior to the diagnosis being made; starting treatment (insulin) may then be associated with weight gain. The individual may experience a rise in concerns about body image following this weight gain, leading, in susceptible individuals, to the onset of eating disorder symptoms. The rigid dietary "rules" that the patient must follow might also serve as a trigger for increasing preoccupation with food choices, composition and calories, potentially progressing to food restriction, or development of compensatory behaviors to undo the effects of foods that have been ingested. In addition, periods of hypoglycemia, activating intense hunger, may be experienced in negative ways, leading either to overeating or restriction out of concern for weight gain. Obesity, a risk factor for type 2 diabetes, may be a consequence of BED or BN and may contribute to low self-esteem and body image concerns which may further the cycle of disordered eating, with any combination of binge eating, restricting, and compensatory behaviors.

Insulin omission, a form of compensatory behavior that Francine is exhibiting, may be particularly common in adolescent

females with type 1 diabetes. Skipping insulin will impair the body's ability to incorporate ingested glucose, such that some of the calories eaten are eliminated. It results in impaired glycemic control, with short- and long-term consequences, including diabetic ketoacidosis and end-organ damage from uncontrolled hyperglycemia (e.g., retinopathy, nephropathy, and cardiovascular disease). The clinician may suspect insulin omission in a patient with diabetes who takes insulin, where there is evidence of worsening glycemic control, weight loss, and recurrent episodes of DKA, in the context of suspicion that the individual may be concerned about body image or weight gain.

Other chronic medical conditions may put vulnerable individuals at increased risk for developing an eating disorder. Autoimmune conditions, for example, requiring chronic corticosteroid use, may contribute to weight gain, leading to concerns about body weight and shape. Endocrine disorders that affect appetite or metabolism may similarly increase preoccupation with food and weight, initiating symptoms of an eating disorder.

6.2.2 Assessment

Francine's evaluation should include further assessment of beliefs and behaviors she may exhibit related to eating and body image. Dr. Green should obtain a full eating history, including past engagement in calorie restriction or binge-eating, as well as compensatory behaviors other than insulin manipulation, such as vomiting, laxative or diuretic use, or excessive exercise. Francine can be encouraged to elaborate on her thoughts regarding her body shape and weight, and their influence on her sense of acceptability and self-worth. She should be screened for depression, which is more common in individuals living with diabetes than in the general population.

6.2.3 Eating Disorders and Online Media

Francine alluded to information she has read online. There exists a sizeable, and dangerous, internet presence that encourages eating disordered behavior. Essays, blog entries, social media, and message boards "educate" readers about ways to lose weight, promote an idealization of extreme thinness, and offer "support" to individuals who are engaging in restricting and compensatory behaviors. Users of these sites and social media may coach and encourage each others' eating disorders. Adolescents, perhaps more than others, may be highly susceptible to the influence of such content; developmentally, they are striving to establish and solidify their identity, searching for sources of self-esteem through "belonging" to an identified group. Individuals with eating disorders may feel particularly isolated and may turn to online content and social media to find support and solidarity, as well as concrete advice.

There is a large and still growing presence of eating disorder-promoting Web sites and content. These sites offer information (much of it misleading or inaccurate) about nutrition and weight loss, with suggestions on ways to restrict and compensate for ingested calories, as well as suggestions on how to hide the signs of the eating disorder from others, such as parents or doctors. The web pages and message boards are full of "tips", such as drinking excessive water to stay "full" and also before being weighed at the doctor's office, keeping a journal of pictures of skinny bodies for "motivation," and ways to facilitate purging. The tone of these sites is, on the surface, supportive and empathic; but the effect on the reader and follower can be frankly malignant. Because of the dangerous nature of such sites—idealizing unhealthy bodies and promoting dangerous behavior—they are often shut down by regulators. To avoid being found and closed, many use disguised language, such as referring to anorexia nervosa as if writing about a person, "Ana". The clinician with some knowledge about such online content may better be able to detect signs and symptoms of an eating disorder in a patient and will be able to address the use of these sites (including the incorrect information and unsafe practices they promote) as part of the patient's treatment [1].

6.3 Differential Diagnosis

The differential diagnosis for a patient with diabetes who is losing weight and persistently hyperglycemic should include inadequate insulin dosing or other physiological reasons for why the prescribed amount of insulin is not being effective. When poor adherence with insulin is suspected, reasons for non-adherence should be considered, such as impaired access to prescription refills, life stressors, or emotional or psychiatric disorders that may be impeding full adherence (such as depression).

When an eating disorder is suspected in such a patient, the various relevant feeding or eating disorders should be reviewed. As noted previously, Francine is not yet substantially underweight, and thus does not meet criteria for AN (though, if left untreated, she might continue to lose weight and would, if other criteria are met, be appropriately diagnosed with AN). She is not binge-eating and therefore does not fit the diagnoses of BN or BED. As the nature of her eating disorder can be described (i.e., she is normal weight, using insulin omission for weight loss), she should not be classified as unspecified feeding or eating disorder.

6.4 Outcome

Addressing Francine's eating disorder will best be accomplished through a true biopsychosocial approach. Her medical and psychiatric issues are indelibly intertwined and linked to the social context in which she lives. Involvement of her endocrinologist and other medical doctors, her psychiatrist, a nutritionist, and her family, will be a key to establishing a foundation upon which Francine can begin to change her behaviors, her experience of food and her body, and her medical care.

Education about the risks of uncontrolled hyperglycemia, in addition to information about the medical and emotional consequences of insulin omission and eating disorders in general, can be offered. Because rigid dietary guidelines may be particularly problematic for an individual with an eating disorder, it may be useful to allow for more flexibility in the patient's approach to

eating and food choices. Nutritional counseling will be an essential part of Francine's treatment. Psychotherapy, such as Cognitive–Behavioral Therapy (CBT), may help her to break the cycle of distorted body beliefs, low self-esteem, and disordered eating. Supportive and psychodynamic psychotherapeutic approaches may allow exploration of Francine's concerns about her body, her health, and her self-worth. Addressing any comorbid psychiatric conditions, such as an anxiety or depressive disorder, is essential.

Engaging the family system is a mainstay of the treatment of feeding or eating disorders in adolescent patients. Family-based therapies have been developed to specifically target eating disorders, involving the family in the individual's treatment, while minimizing detrimental patterns of behavior within the family that may worsen the situation [2].

Francine was highly reluctant to admit to any misuse or omission of insulin, and even more resistant to speaking about her eating and her thoughts about her body and shape. Her parents reported to Dr. Green that she continued to spend all of her time on her computer or phone and became tearful or angry around any conversations about her diabetes, as well as at most mealtimes. Dr. Green referred Francine and her parents to a colleague with an expertise in family therapy for adolescents with AN (the Maudsley approach) and an individual therapist. She began working with a nutritionist whom she really liked—someone who used phone apps and other technology to engage Francine about her food choices and tracking. In individual therapy, Francine became less guarded and began talking more about her experience of living with diabetes—from frustration to fear—as well as her anxieties about the future, most notably her worries about leaving home for college ("I always used to think I was such an independent person, but I also sometimes think that I might fall apart without them... what will happen to me?"). With time, her parents and providers (as well as Francine, herself), noted improved communication at home, and less conflict around eating and diabetes management. Her glycemic control improved, and her weight stabilized. She appeared happier and more engaged with her family, and, ultimately, more self-assured and grown-up.

References

1. Harshbarger JL, Ahlers-Schmidt CR, Mayans L, Mayans D, Hawkins JH. Pro-anorexia websites: what a clinician should know. Int J Eat Disord. 2009;42:367–70.
2. Smith A, Cook-Cottone C. A review of family therapy as an effective intervention for anorexia nervosa in adolescents. Psychol Med Settings. 2011;18:323–34.

Suggested Reading

Pinhas-Hamiel O, Levy-Shraga Y. Eating disorders in adolescents with type 2 and type 1 diabetes. Curr Diab Rep. 2013;13:289–97.

Part II
Patients who Eat Too Much

Chapter 7
Ginny, the Secret Eater

7.1 Case Presentation

Ginny, a 23-year-old woman enrolled in a Masters of Fine Arts program, presents to see Dr. Hamilton for an initial assessment for an outpatient eating disorder program, after seeking help at her student health program with symptoms of persistent overeating and self-induced vomiting. Ginny tells Dr. Hamilton that food has "always been a problem" for her; she recalls spending afternoons after school eating a box of cookies or crackers while watching television, or turning to food when she felt "upset." Overweight as a child, she became increasingly self-conscious about her weight in adolescence, and at age 14, she began dieting excessively, substantially reducing her calorie intake and losing approximately 20 lb in two months, and then continuing to lose weight, causing concern in her parents and teachers. She began seeing a therapist and a nutritionist and was slowly able to normalize her eating patterns and to maintain a healthy weight for the rest of high school, though continuing to count calories and weigh herself daily, with heightened anxiety and brief periods of food restriction in response to any fluctuations in her weight. At the end of her first year of college, after gaining several pounds over the year, she began restricting her food intake more consistently, going on a

© Springer International Publishing Switzerland 2017
J. Gordon-Elliott, *Fundamentals of Diagnosing and Treating
Eating Disorders*, DOI 10.1007/978-3-319-46065-9_7

"crash diet" of approximately 800 kilocalories per day. During the examination period, having difficulty concentrating on her work and under stress, she began eating large amounts of food beginning at about 9 p.m., such as 5 slices of pizza, or a box of cereal and a pint of ice cream. After returning home for the summer, she tried to normalize her eating, but continued to eat at night in a way that felt "out of control" and one night caused herself to vomit, so distressed by how much she had eaten. Over the course of the summer, a pattern developed of excessive eating followed by self-induced vomiting approximately twice a week. She continued this upon her return to school, becoming increasingly avoidant of social eating situations and progressively isolating from friends. She could periodically stop the vomiting, but anxiety about her weight and feeling unable to control her eating would lead to recurrence of vomiting. She began trying laxatives on occasion to try to eliminate calories without needing to vomit, though continued to vomit as well. During her first year of graduate school, with more unstructured academic time and adjusting to a new city without her usual social supports, her bingeing and purging behavior increased. By the time she presented to student health, she was engaging in this five times a week, on average, sometimes twice in a day.

She currently endorses low mood and significant anxiety "all the time," with most of her thoughts focusing on her food and weight. She denies excessive exercise or use of any pills other than occasional laxative use. She reports minimal alcohol use and denies illicit substance use. Her BMI is 26, weighing 147 lb at 5′3″.

7.2 Diagnosis/Assessment

Preferred diagnosis: Bulimia Nervosa

Bulimia Nervosa (BN) is characterized by a pattern of binge eating, associated with compensatory behavior to prevent weight gain, and an undue influence of body shape and weight on the individual's feelings about her/himself [see Text Box: Bulimia Nervosa: Terminology; see Text Box: Bulimia Nervosa: DSM-5 Diagnostic Criteria].

Bulimia Nervosa: Terminology

What defines an episode of *binge eating*?

The DSM defines binge eating as (BOTH):

- Eating in a discrete amount of time large amounts of food.
- A sense of lack of control over eating during an episode.

Binge eating behavior may take many forms, but there are some features that may be more typical. Binges are most commonly preceded by negative emotions and may lead to a brief sense of relief or emotional numbing. Some will report feeling in a dissociated state during the binge. Binges may be experienced by the individual as impulsive, or they may be planned. The binge often involves food that the individual would normally avoid, and there is commonly a sense of shame over the behavior and efforts to conceal. The time frame of the binge may vary, but should occur over a limited period of time (generally within 2 hours); "grazing" or eating smaller amounts of food that cumulatively contribute to an excess of calories over the day would *not* constitute a binge.

What constitutes *inappropriate compensatory behaviors*?

The most commonly used purging behavior is volitional vomiting. This typically follows a large-volume binge, but in some individuals, vomiting may be used after smaller amounts of food intake, as well. Other purging behaviors may include use of laxatives, enemas, or diuretics. Additional behaviors, not traditionally considered *purging* methods, may be used to "undo" calorie intake, such as excessive exercise or calorie restriction; less commonly, individuals may take medication with the intent of increasing the metabolic rate (such as stimulants or inappropriate thyroid hormone use), and patients with type I diabetes may manipulate their use of insulin to limit glucose absorption [see Chap. 6].

Bulimia Nervosa: DSM-5 Diagnostic Criteria

- Recurrent episodes of binge eating
- Recurrent inappropriate compensatory behavior in order to prevent weight gain (purging).

- The binge eating and compensatory behaviors both occur, on average, at least once a week for three months.
- Self-evaluation is unduly influenced by body shape and weight.
- The disturbance does not occur exclusively during episodes of anorexia nervosa.

7.2.1 Clinical Features

Ginny's presentation is typical for individuals with BN. Her symptoms include recurrent binge eating episodes, at least once a week, in which she eats more food during a short period of time than would be considered normal, with a sense of loss of control over her eating during the episodes; she engages in compensatory behaviors, including vomiting and laxative use, as well as some periods of calorie restriction; her self-esteem and body image are tightly and inextricably linked. Her history, characteristic of many with BN, is notable for a long-standing pattern of preoccupation with food and body shape/weight, and a progression of eating disorder symptoms over time. Individuals with BN will commonly describe an earlier period of food restriction without binge eating or compensatory behavior; over time, prolonged calorie restriction or a sense of deprivation will stimulate episodes of binge eating which then—due to concern about weight gain—lead to experimentation with, followed by recurrent engagement in, purging behavior, such as self-induced vomiting.

Individuals with BN are typically normal weight or moderately overweight (BMI between 18.5 and 30), as purging behaviors after binges do not sufficiently compensate for calorie intake. Most commonly, BN develops in late adolescence or early adulthood. The prevalence in North American and European samples is in the range of 0.5–1.5 %, with a substantial female to male predominance. The natural course of the illness is for symptoms to diminish over time, though in many there may develop a chronic course,

with or without periods of remission and relapse. There may be ongoing shift in symptoms over time, in any order, from a predominance of binge eating and compensatory behaviors, to a pattern of food restriction, to binge eating without compensatory behaviors. Individuals may fulfill criteria for distinct feeding or eating disorders at different points in their course of symptomatic illness [see *Differential Diagnosis* for more discussion].

BN carries significant medical risk, with a substantially increased all-cause mortality rate compared to the general population, related to a combination of medical consequences, psychiatric comorbidity, and suicide. The more serious medical complications of BN include electrolyte disturbances leading to cardiac conduction abnormalities and seizures; esophageal and gastric tears (even rupture in severe cases) and upper gastrointestinal bleeding; pancreatitis; aspiration pneumonitis; and patients who ingest ipecac syrup in order to induce vomiting may develop life-threatening sequelae including cardiac myopathies and damage to skeletal muscle throughout the body [2].

7.2.2 Comorbidity

Overlap with other psychiatric conditions is the norm rather than the exception in individuals with BN. There appears to be an increased frequency of depressive disorders, bipolar and related disorders, post-traumatic stress disorder, anxiety disorders, and personality disorders. Substance use disorders may co-occur in up to one-third of patients. Suicide is several times more common for those with a diagnosis of BN compared to the general population, and more than one-quarter of individuals with BN may attempt suicide at some point [see Chap. 8 for further discussion of comorbidity in BN].

7.2.3 Assessment

The initial safety assessment of individuals with BN should include evaluation of safety, including medical and psychiatric factors.

Patients with any concerns for the more serious medical complications of the disorder, such as upper gastrointestinal bleeding or cardiac arrhythmia, should be referred for emergency medical attention. Suicidal thoughts or behaviors, non-suicidal self-harming behaviors, and substance use should be screened for immediately, with referral to hospital-level care if there are concerns for imminent risk of harm.

The general medical review of systems may reveal complaints of gastric reflux, and sensations of bloating or early satiety as well as constipation; patients may describe weakness and dizziness, as well as palpitations; menstrual abnormalities are also common. The physical evaluation, which can be done in conjunction with the patient's medical provider, will include measuring height, weight, and vital signs, performing a physical examination, and obtaining basic laboratory studies as well as an electrocardiogram if there are concerns for cardiac abnormalities. The assessment may reveal hypotension and tachycardia; hyponatremia and hypokalemia; visibly evident parotid gland enlargement; erosion of dental enamel with evidence of dental caries or decay; and edema and dry skin. Russell's sign is the presence of scarring or a callus on the dorsum of the hand due to using one's fingers for self-induced vomiting.

The assessment should include a review of current eating behaviors, including current patterns of binge eating and compensatory behaviors; inquiry into any eating rituals or "rules" the individual may have established (such as rigidity regarding food choices, or when or in what situations the patient is "allowed" to eat, order in which food items are consumed, etc.); and a full screen for past eating disorders, as well as disordered patterns of eating that may not have fulfilled criteria for a feeding or eating disorder. The impact of food, body weight, and body image on self-esteem, mental state, and functioning should be explored. Screening tools, such as the five-item self-report measure SCOFF [see Chap. 3 for more information on screening tools], can be utilized. A full psychiatric evaluation, including past or current co-occurring psychiatric disorders [see *Comorbidity* and *Differential Diagnosis*], is important.

7.2.4   Treatment

Once the diagnosis of BN has been made and urgent medical and safety issues have been addressed, treatment may include psychotherapy, nutritional rehabilitation, and pharmacotherapy, with the combination of all three demonstrating the best outcomes. Normalization of eating and food-related behaviors is the foundation of initial treatment. A regular eating routine should be instituted (e.g., three meals and two snacks at determined times of the day), with safeguards implemented to minimize the risk of compensatory behaviors (e.g., no access to bathrooms for a period of time after eating). Nutritional education may be useful for some individuals. Cognitive Behavioral Therapy (CBT) may help in a variety of ways—from developing a structured eating schedule, to integrating new activities and behaviors that can distract from or replace maladaptive eating-related behaviors, to addressing some of the dysfunctional thoughts and negative emotions that may perpetuate the eating disorder. Though less well studied, Dialectical Behavioral Therapy (DBT) may also be effective in this population, whether or not there is a co-occurring personality disorder [1, 5].

Pharmacotherapy has been found to be effective in the treatment in BN, though less effective on its own than psychotherapy alone. First-line treatment is fluoxetine with a target dose of 60 mg. Fluoxetine is supported by the most evidence, demonstrating improvement in the core symptoms of BN of binge eating and purging behavior, as well as reduction in preoccupation with food and body dissatisfaction. Second-line treatment would include other selective serotonin reuptake inhibitors (SSRIs); they have been shown to be effective in the treatment of BN, but with fewer studies to support their use. Beyond these options, clinicians might consider other antidepressants, such as serotonin norepinephrine reuptake inhibitors (SNRIs), and tricyclic antidepressants; there is also some evidence for the use of topiramate. Bupropion should be avoided as it may increase the risk for seizures, which patients with BN may be predisposed to due to electrolyte abnormalities as a consequence of vomiting and other compensatory behaviors [3].

Long-term treatment may involve a combination of medication and psychotherapy to address relapse prevention and treat any

comorbid psychiatric conditions. Self-report measures can be used to track symptoms and illness severity over time, such as the Bulimia Test-Revised (BULIT-R) and the Eating Disorder Examination-Questionnaire (EDE-Q). Computer-based tracking programs, such as phone apps and logs, may be useful in engaging patients in monitoring symptoms over time and may facilitate reporting of symptoms and communication between patient and clinician [4].

Spotlight on DSM-5: Bulimia Nervosa
The diagnostic criteria for BN in DSM-5 are largely unchanged from DSM-IV. The frequency of required episodes of binge eating/compensatory behavior decreased from twice a week in DSM-IV-TR to once a week in DSM-5 because of the lack of clinically meaningful differences between individuals who display these symptoms once a week compared to twice or more times a week. Additionally, there was removal of the subtypes (purging and nonpurging types); all patients with bulimia must engage in some compensatory behavior, and it was not determined to be useful to divide patients up based on whether they used purging methods such as vomiting, laxative use, and diuretics, for example, or other methods, such as fasting or excessive exercise. Lastly, specifiers indicating level of severity (based on the frequency of compensatory behaviors) and remission status were added.

7.3   Differential Diagnosis

As mentioned above, it is not uncommon for eating-related symptoms to vary and fluctuate over time such that there may be a predominance of different features at distinct times, with the individual fulfilling criteria for a different feeding and eating disorder at separate points of illness. This phenomenon, as well as some of the overlapping features of the major disorders in this category, can lead to some ambiguity or diagnostic confusion when

evaluating a patient presenting with symptoms suggestive of an eating disorder [see Text Box: "Focus on Differential Diagnosis"].

The diagnosis of BN emphasizes the two core features of binge eating and compensatory behaviors to "undo" the binges. BN is distinguished from the other disorder that involves prominent binge eating, binge eating disorder [BED (see Chap. 9 for further discussion)], most notably by the presence of the compensatory behaviors, which should be absent in BED. Other features may be different in individuals with BN compared to those with BED, such as weight (typically patients with BN are normal to somewhat overweight, while those with BED are overweight), but weight is not a criterion of either—the diagnoses must be differentiated based on whether or not there are prominent compensatory behaviors.

BN shares one central feature with the other major feeding or eating disorder, anorexia nervosa (AN), that distinguishes them, conceptually, from the other disorders: an intense preoccupation with body image that ostensibly drives the other core behaviors of each disorder. BN differs from AN, however, not by what is *present* in BN but by what is *absent*—namely, the core feature of AN of persistent behaviors that maintain a significantly low weight. As soon as this feature is identified, whether or not there is binge eating or purging (which are present, though usually the volume of binge eating is less, in the *Binge Eating/Purging Type* of AN), the diagnosis of AN should be the primary one to consider. The clinician should then further investigate whether the patient exhibits the other features of AN, including intense fear of weight gain or refusal to gain weight [which would differentiate AN from another eating disorder that may be characterized by a very low weight, such as avoidant/restrictive food intake disorder, in which the driving force is thought to be unrelated to body image or a desire for thinness (ARFID; see Chaps. 1 and 4 for further discussion of AN and ARFID)].

In addition to the other core feeding or eating disorders, the diagnostic evaluation should include consideration of additional disorders which may present with prominent eating-related

symptoms. Overeating may be present in major depressive disorder, as well as additional psychiatric disorders with prominent impulsivity, such as borderline personality disorder; medical conditions with hyperphagia include Prader–Willi syndrome and Klein-Levin syndrome. The presence of compensatory behaviors, however, is not a feature of these disorders.

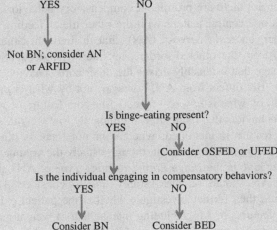

Focus on Differential Diagnosis: General Approach to an Eating Disorder Presentation

Is the individual significantly low-weight with behaviors preventing weight gain?
                YES   NO

                                        Not BN; consider AN
                                             or ARFID

                                        Is binge-eating present?
                                        YES   NO

                                                Consider OSFED or UFED

                        Is the individual engaging in compensatory behaviors?
                        YES   NO

                        Consider BN   Consider BED

AN   anorexia nervosa
BN   bulimia nervosa
BED   binge eating disorder
OSFED   other specified feeding or eating disorder
UFED   unspecified feeding or eating disorder

7.4 Outcome

Ginny is presenting to Dr. Hamilton with motivation to address her symptoms. Numerous factors—including, but not limited to, anxiety about relinquishing symptoms, shame about one's behaviors, impaired insight, and comorbid psychiatric conditions—may delay help-seeking in individuals with eating disorders and make the treatment more challenging. As the distress related to the symptoms or consequences of the eating behavior rises, motivation to change may increase. In Ginny's case, her symptoms are becoming harder for her to tolerate—essentially, the "advantages" of her behaviors (e.g., her perceived control over her weight and body, or any temporary reduction in negative emotional states that she experiences either from the binging or the purging) are beginning to no longer outweigh their disadvantages (e.g., shame, isolation, or negative consequences on her health and functioning), and she is beginning to experience the motivation to change.

Dr. Hamilton will want to capitalize on this motivation, encouraging the part of Ginny that is looking for a way out of her symptoms, while outlining a clear plan of action. A nonjudgmental and knowledgeable stance can be useful when engaging patients with eating disorders, because of the combination of shame about their behaviors and ambivalence about giving up symptoms that is so commonly present. After a full psychiatric history and screening for comorbid conditions, Dr. Hamilton begins by summarizing back to Ginny what she is identifying as negative consequences of her illness, while validating how challenging it must be to seek help and consider change. He then provides psychoeducation about the risks of BN (medical and psychological) and lays out a preliminary plan of treatment. He recommends that she enter an eating disorder day program where she will participate in nutritional counseling, group therapy, and behavioral interventions (e.g., two meals a day at the program with prevention of purging after meals). He acknowledges the anxiety that she describes feeling and suggests a trial of fluoxetine to address anxiety and eating disorder; she begins at 20 mg daily with the plan to increase as indicated.

After six weeks at the program full time, she is able to transition to weekly meetings with Dr. Hamilton and biweekly nutritionist

visits. She finds it harder to avoid bingeing on weekends and has developed a plan whereby she keeps herself occupied with social activities after dinner on weekend nights to prevent purging, which in turn reduces her likelihood to binge. She is reassured to see that her weight does not increase, though she remains worried about this and can sense in herself an urge to restrict calories, which she talks about in her therapy. She understands that she is at risk of relapse in the short and long term, but is hopeful that the sense of accomplishment she has gained from curbing her symptoms—as well as the emotional and social benefits she has noted since addressing her symptoms—will keep her invested in her treatment and vigilant to not slipping back into the disorder.

References

1. Kass AE, Kolko RP, Wilfley DE. Psychological treatments for eating disorders. Curr Opin Psychiatry. 2013;26:549–55.
2. Mitchell JE, Crow S. Medical complications of anorexia nervosa and bulimia nervosa. Curr Opin Psychiatry. 2006;19:438–43.
3. Mitchell JE, Roerig J, Steffen K. Biological therapies for eating disorders. Int J Eat Disord. 2013;46:470–7.
4. Peterson CB, Mitchell JE. Self-report measures. In: Mitchell JE, Peterson CB, editors. Assessment of eating disorders. New York: Guilford Publications; 2005. p. 98.
5. Wisniewski L, Ben-Porath DD. Dialectical behavior therapy and eating disorders: the use of contingency management procedures to manage dialectical dilemmas. Am J Psychother. 2015;69:129–40.

Suggested Readings

Bakalar JL, Shank LM, Vannucci A, Radin RM, Tanofsky-Kraff MT. Recent advances in development and risk factor research on eating disorders. Curr Psychiatry Rep. 2015;17:42.
Mehler PS, Anderson AE. Eating disorders: a guide to medical care and complications. 2nd ed. Baltimore: The Johns Hopkins University Press; 2010.

Chapter 8
Hannah's Troubles

8.1 Case Presentation

Hannah is a 28-year-old single woman who presents to Dr. Ingram for an initial psychiatric appointment with a chief complaint of "I have binge eating disorder and I think I might benefit from the medication I saw on the commercial." Hannah reports to Dr. Ingram a 15-year history of episodes of overeating (sometimes only having a second portion of food, but other times eating large quantities of food such as two boxes of cookies and a pint of ice cream). She describes feeling unable to stop until she feels "so full" she needs to vomit. She states that she does this on average once a week, though has periods where it is more or less frequent. She denies misusing laxatives or exercise for weight control. She will sometimes restrict her food intake for a couple of days in a row, eating approximately 500 calories per day, in order to "make up" for her overeating or if she is "feeling bloated." She is 5'7" and 130 lb, with a BMI of 20.4. She reports that her eating episodes are typically triggered by feeling angry or upset with others, such as her boyfriend, Tom.

She also reports drinking "several" alcoholic drinks three nights a week "with friends"; she is hesitant to further quantify, but admits that she does occasionally have loss of memory of events

© Springer International Publishing Switzerland 2017   75
J. Gordon-Elliott, *Fundamentals of Diagnosing and Treating
Eating Disorders*, DOI 10.1007/978-3-319-46065-9_8

during a period of intoxication and explains this has "caused" her to do "stupid things," such as having sexual encounters with men other than Tom, which has caused problems in their relationship. She has never tried to stop drinking and has never sought treatment for it. She reports erratic sleep patterns, with some weekends where she only sleeps 2–3 h a night, but then will have to take off a day from work the next week to sleep. She admits to having difficulty with "frustration" and will "scratch" her skin with her fingernails in response to such emotions, sometimes drawing blood. She relates one psychiatric hospitalization at age 13 after she disclosed to her school counselor that she had cut her outer forearm with a razor blade (no sutures needed) and taken 5 tablets of acetaminophen earlier that day. She believes she was given a diagnosis of "depression" at the time. She has occasionally been to therapists and psychiatrists and says she has been told she is "depressed" or "bipolar," with past short trials of fluoxetine, sertraline, lamotrigine, topiramate, and risperidone. She never continued any of the medications for more than a few weeks, due to not feeling they were helpful or because of side effects.

When Dr. Ingram asks what Hannah hopes will be different this time in treatment, she states that she hears that the medication lisdexamfetamine (Vyvanse) can help stop binge eating disorder, and she would like to try it.

8.2 Diagnosis/Assessment

Preferred diagnosis: Alcohol Use Disorder. Bulimia nervosa.

8.3 Differential Diagnosis

The case of Hannah highlights the complexity of psychiatric diagnosis. Even in relatively straightforward situations, there can be uncertainty about whether adequate diagnostic criteria are met, and whether a syndrome exceeds the threshold at which it should be considered worthy of clinical attention. More challenging cases, like Hannah's, involve numerous symptoms crossing various

diagnostic categories. The clinician may be left puzzled and unclear about which aspects of the presentation and history to focus on and how to conceptualize the patient's problems. This may result in the clinician overzealously assigning several diagnoses at once, and then potentially not knowing how to prioritize treatment; alternatively, it may lead to overlooking important symptoms or diagnostic clues because of the multitude of information, and assigning a single diagnosis, missing major areas of psychopathology that would benefit from treatment. There exists a constant tension between appropriately assigning diagnoses where criteria are met and following the law of parsimony by explaining a patient's symptoms with as few diagnoses as possible.

Hannah describes frequent binge eating episodes, in which she feels "out of control" with respect to her eating, as well as compensatory activities. These occur on average at least once a week and have been going on for more than three months. Dr. Ingram would want to further tease out the extent to which her body image influences her self-esteem and well-being. If significantly so, she would fulfill criteria for bulimia nervosa (BN). The diagnosis of binge eating disorder (BED) would not be suitable as she does engage in compensatory behaviors; a patient with BED does not. In addition, Hannah most likely has an alcohol use disorder (AUD), with binge drinking episodes which she continues to engage in despite negative consequences on relationships and work, as well as involvement in unsafe behaviors. She reports a history of mood symptoms as well as past "diagnoses" given by other providers including "depression" and "bipolar." Her history of risky and impulsive behaviors, including sexual encounters with men other than her partner and her drinking, as well as her vague reports of sleep disturbance, raises the important question of whether she might indeed have bipolar disorder. Further questioning would be warranted to clarify the duration of her episodes of reduced sleep and whether these also correlate with changes in mood and activity; past depressive episodes would also need to be further explored, to ascertain whether she ever experienced a full major depressive episode. Given her use of alcohol over many years, it might be difficult to confidently diagnose a primary bipolar disorder, though this would be valuable to determine as best as possible. Lastly, there are substantial clues in her history that she has traits of, if not the full-criteria syndrome of, borderline personality disorder

(BPD); her story is notable for evidence of impulsivity, chaotic interpersonal relationships, mood dysregulation and anger, self-injury, and suicidality, all suggesting a diagnosis of BPD.

The question remains: What is Hannah's diagnosis? One could argue that this is a purely academic discussion, and not necessary for clinical management. On the other hand, diagnosis will guide appropriate treatment, and therefore, a firm diagnostic formulation is an essential aspect of clinical care.

There are several ways to approach these kinds of diagnostic challenges. The first step, regardless of one's approach, would be to review the criteria of the various diagnoses to ensure that they do not include any exclusionary conditions to guide the clinician in cases of such diagnostic overlap. For example, as discussed in Chap. 2, the diagnosis of body dysmorphic disorder should not be made if the preoccupation with one's body is better explained by concern with body weight in the context of anorexia nervosa [see Chap. 2 for further discussion about body dysmorphic disorder]. In Hannah's case, in reviewing the various diagnoses we are considering there are no criteria that would automatically rule out one diagnosis over another—she could, theoretically, have all of the above diagnoses.

The next step would be to see whether there is any evidence to guide the clinician about what to do in such cases—i.e., is there an established literature about the co-occurrence of any of the disorders we are considering, or are there any expert consensus statements about how to prioritize a differential diagnosis when the above diagnoses are being considered? In Hannah's case, we know that BN may frequently co-occur with the other diagnoses we are considering. BN and substance use disorders (SUDs) share many core features, including repeated engagement in unhealthy behaviors and impaired ability to inhibit them; some patients with BN will describe an "addictive" quality of the binges. Comorbidity of BN and SUD may be as high as 25 % of individuals with either disorder [4]. Though they may have separate etiologies, these disorders may share common risk factors [6]. BPD and BN also commonly co-occur, with up to a third of individuals with BN also receiving a diagnosis of BPD [2]. They may share modifying risk factors, such as early life trauma, and have features in common, including impulsivity and emotional dysregulation, with engagement in maladaptive behaviors in response to negative emotions

[5]. Patients with BN also have higher rates of bipolar spectrum disorders and depressive disorders than the general population [1, 3].

Once the diagnostic criteria and relevant literature have been adequately reviewed, there still remains the question of which diagnoses are worth formally making, and how inclusive or exclusive the clinician should aim to be. This is where clinicians may differ significantly in terms of their approach. One viewpoint might be that it is best to focus, at least at first, on the disorders that are modifiable (and potentially "reversible"). Another approach might be to concentrate on the diagnoses for which there is the largest evidence base for treatment to guide the clinician. Prioritizing safety is a core principle of medical practice, and it is therefore perhaps the most prudent option to first emphasize the symptoms and associated diagnoses that put the patient most imminently at risk. Lastly, some clinicians might favor identifying problem symptoms and letting those guide treatment, rather than differentiating among various discrete diagnoses.

There are arguments favoring and challenging these alternate approaches. Being parsimonious by simplifying a multifaceted case into one diagnosis will limit competing treatment plans and, potentially, also polypharmacy; on the other hand, such an approach might miss major areas of psychopathology or problematic symptoms. Remaining broad and assigning multiple diagnoses as long as criteria are met may help highlight the numerous issues the patient is struggling with, but could potentially be overlooking the core psychopathology that is driving many of the symptoms. As an example, a patient with BPD may engage in substance use and binge-eating and purging as a function of her impulsivity, which also plays out in her interpersonal relationships and her self-injurious behavior. Being able to conceptualize symptoms across diagnoses as being related to specific deficits or difficulties a patient has can allow for focused treatment that can target some of the more problematic symptoms, rather than adding a new treatment modality for each distinct diagnosis.

Whether being guided by diagnostic categories or by symptom clusters, it is recommended—especially in more complex cases—that the clinician routinely reassess the situation and question initial

assumptions: Is there something that is being missed?; Is there a single diagnosis, or perhaps just one or two, that would explain the multitude of symptoms?; Is there a whole area of psychopathology that is being ignored?

8.4 Outcome

Dr. Ingram learned more about Hannah's difficulties over the course of three sessions. He was able to rule out with fair confidence a bipolar spectrum disorder. Hannah was able to better elaborate on her alcohol use, and though it was clearly a problematic symptom, it appeared to be a less frequent behavior than initially suggested; notably, it was identified that her binge-drinking would typically occur after an interpersonal dispute. Dr. Ingram was able to identify long-standing disordered eating patterns and more substantial bulimic symptoms than what Hannah had initially admitted to, including daily engagement in behaviors such as purging, spitting out of chewed food, and laxative use, which she had initially denied. Hannah disclosed other self-injurious behavior, including head-banging and occasional skin-burning, as well as severe anxiety and emotional distress related to interpersonal insecurities and threat of loss of attachment figures.

Dr. Ingram conceptualized Hannah as having borderline personality disorder as well as bulimia nervosa. Because of the frequency of her bulimic symptoms and the physical risks she was putting herself in through these behaviors, Dr. Ingram prioritized treatment of her eating disorder. She agreed to engage in an eating disorder outpatient program which used principles of dialectial behavioral therapy (DBT). Dr. Ingram initiated fluoxetine with the goal of improvement of BN symptoms and potentially also the impulsivity that seemed to drive her various problematic behaviors and her interpersonal difficulties. As alcohol had tended to worsen her symptoms of bingeing, Hannah was counseled about minimizing this behavior, which she was amenable to because she was increasingly invested in stopping her bingeing and purging (finding it to be more of a hindrance in her life than a something that she felt she wanted to engage in anymore). With improvement in her eating

disorder, she was shifted over to the primary DBT program at the same center, where she worked with her treatment team on reducing self-injurious behaviors and learning to self-regulate her mood. No further medications were added.

References

1. Campos RN, Dos Santos DJ, Cordás TA, Angst J, Moreno RA. Occurrence of bipolar spectrum disorder and comorbidities in women with eating disorders. Int J Bipolar Disord. 2013;1:25.
2. Cassin SE, von Ranson KM. Personality and eating disorders: a decade in review. Clin Psychol Rev. 2005;25:895–916.
3. Godart NT, Perdereau F, Rein Z, Berthoz S, Wallier J, Jeammet P, et al. Comorbidity studies of eating disorders and mood disorders: Critical review of the literature. J Affect Disord. 2007;97:37–49.
4. Holderness CC, Brooks-Gunn J, Warren MP. Co-morbidity of eating disorders and substance abuse review of the literature. Int J Eat Disord. 1994;16:1–34.
5. Selby EA, Doyle P, Crosby RD, Wonderlich SA, Engel SG, Mitchell JD, Le Grange D. Momentary emotion surrounding bulimic behaviors in women with bulimia nervosa and borderline personality disorder. J Psychiatr Res. 2012;46(11):1492–500.
6. Stice E, Burton EM, Shaw H. Prospective relations between bulimic pathology, depression, and substance abuse: Unpacking comorbidity in adolescent girls. J Consult Clin Psychol. 2004;72:62–71.

Suggested Readings

Davis C. A narrative review of binge eating and addictive behaviors: shared associations with seasonality and personality factors. Front Psychiatry. 2013;4:183.
Godt K. Personality disorders in 545 patients with eating disorders. Eur Eat Disord Rev. 2008;16:94–9.
Sysko R, Hildebrandt T. Cognitive-behavioural therapy for individuals with bulimia nervosa and a Co-occurring substance use disorder. Eur Eat Disord Rev. 2009;17(2):89–100.

Chapter 9
Ian, the Guilty Eater

9.1 Case Presentation

Ian is a 41-year-old married father of three, who is referred to psychiatrist, Dr. Jarvis, by his internist, Dr. Tang, for evaluation of depression. Ian had not been receiving routine medical care until he turned 40, when he started seeing Dr. Tang as part of his health evaluation for life insurance. Noted at the time to be in the obese range (weight 210 lb, height 5′9″; BMI 31), Dr. Tang suggested that he lose weight, with some general counseling on weight management and nutritional advice given. Over the following year, despite reporting he wanted to lose weight, Ian's weight increased to 218 lb. He admits to Dr. Tang that he feels demoralized by this and embarrassed about not being able to lose the weight, despite her recommendation that he do so—"I'm a Type A guy; if there's something I need to do, I make it happen!"

On evaluation, Ian reports to Dr. Jarvis that he does not think he has ever had mood issues in the past. He reports being very satisfied overall with his life, including his happy marriage of 13 years, his 3 healthy children, and his career as a financial planner at a major bank. He explains that he maintained a stable weight of 180 lb in his 20s and early 30s, but his weight began increasing over the past several years in the context of increasing

© Springer International Publishing Switzerland 2017   83
J. Gordon-Elliott, *Fundamentals of Diagnosing and Treating
Eating Disorders*, DOI 10.1007/978-3-319-46065-9_9

pressures at home and work. He describes a reasonable diet for most of the day, most days of the week, though with heavy "fast-food" lunches at work; he has been exercising less consistently. When Dr. Jarvis asks more about how his mood and "stress" may be influencing his eating, Ian admits that one or two times a week, he will go down to the kitchen after his wife is in bed and eat all the leftovers from dinner, or perhaps several bowls of the kids' cereal or a bag or 2 of chips. He reluctantly describes these episodes—"I eat so quickly, like I need the food to disappear fast before my wife catches me... I'm not even sure I taste it!" He reports regretting his eating afterward and waking up the next morning feeling angry with himself. He denies ever compensating for the eating by substantially restricting his calories the next day, or engaging in vomiting, laxative use, or excessive exercise.

9.2 Diagnosis/Assessment

Preferred diagnosis: Binge Eating Disorder

The diagnosis of binge eating disorder (BED) is made when an individual is engaging in at least one binge eating episode per week, accompanied by negative physical and emotional responses (such as feeling uncomfortably full, or shame about the eating), without recurrent compensatory behavior [see Chap. 7, Text Box: Bulimia Nervosa: Terminology], and the symptoms have persisted for at least three months and are causing distress or functional impairment. Specifiers are used to document the degree of remission, if present, as well as the severity of the symptoms. A new addition to the Feeding or Eating Disorders chapter in DSM-5, BED intends to describe a discrete syndrome of dysfunctional eating behavior with physical and psychological consequences worthy of psychiatric attention [see Text box: Binge Eating Disorder: DSM-5 Diagnostic Criteria; see Text box: Spotlight on DSM-5: Binge Eating Disorder].

Binge Eating Disorder: DSM-5 Diagnostic Criteria

A. Recurrent episodes of binge eating
B. The binge-eating episodes are associated with three (or more) of the following:

1. Eating much more rapidly than normal.
2. Eating until feeling uncomfortably full.
3. Eating large amounts of food when not feeling physically hungry.
4. Eating alone because of feeling embarrassed by how much one is eating.
5. Feeling disgusted with oneself, depressed, or very guilty afterward.

C. Marked distress regarding binge eating is present.
D. The binge eating occurs, on average, at least once a week for 3 months.
E. The binge eating is not associated with the recurrent use of inappropriate compensatory behavior as in bulimia nervosa and does not occur exclusively during the course of bulimia nervosa or anorexia nervosa.

Specify if:

In partial remission: After full criteria for binge-eating disorder were previously met, binge eating occurs at an average frequency of less than one episode per week for a sustained period of time.

In full remission: After full criteria for binge-eating disorder were previously met, none of the criteria have been met for a sustained period of time.

Specify current severity:

Mild: 1–3 binge eating episodes per week.
Moderate: 4–7 binge eating episodes per week.
Severe: 8–13 binge eating episodes per week.
Extreme: 14 or more binge eating episodes per week.

Spotlight on DSM-5: Binge Eating Disorder

Originally appearing as a variant of bulimia nervosa in DSM-III, BED was first identified as a separate entity in DSM-IV, located in Appendix B (Criteria Sets and Axes Provided for Further Study). Prior to DSM-5, when it was moved into the Feeding or Eating Disorders chapter, patients fulfilling the criteria for binge eating disorder were given a diagnosis of eating disorder not otherwise specified (ED-NOS). The inclusion of BED into the Feeding or Eating Disorders chapter brings the disorder into a central location with other similar conditions; this update also allows more specificity in diagnosing individuals with eating-related conditions, with fewer patients being given the overly broad diagnosis of ED-NOS.

The diagnostic criteria for BED were largely maintained in the transition from DSM-IV to DSM-5; modifications included reduction in the required frequency of binge eating episodes from twice to once a week and the duration of symptoms from six months to three months. These changes reflect the updated appreciation that these cutoffs identify the point at which a clinically meaningful problem is present.

Distinct from a pattern of overeating (i.e., ingesting more calories than are utilized by the body, either on a daily or on an occasional basis), the diagnosis of BED was developed in order to identify a behavioral pattern with clinical significance—not just a "lack of willpower," but a disorder that warrants evaluation and treatment. Many individuals frequently overeat, but in BED there are discrete binge episodes associated with a loss of control and associated distress and impairment. A binge in BED is defined in the same way as it is for bulimia nervosa (BN) [see Chap. 7, Text Box: Bulimia Nervosa: Terminology]. What characterizes a binge for one person will be different from another, depending on the factors such as body size, metabolic needs, and usual patterns of eating. Patients with BED binge-eat at least once a week. The binge is experienced as a negative experience, with diagnostic criteria requiring some combination of emotional and physical distress such as shame, guilt, or a feeling of eating despite being uncomfortably full. Different from BN, patients with BED do not

engage in recurrent compensatory behaviors, such as vomiting or calorie restriction. The binge episode, itself, is similar in BED and BN, but the explicit inclusion of associated emotional/physical disturbing symptoms is unique to BED. The requirement of these additional features, as well as the criterion that marked distress regarding the binge is present, intend to more clearly distinguish BED from a less pathological pattern of overeating that would not be considered a diagnosable disorder.

Patients with BED may eat normally outside of the binge episodes. They may binge-eat in isolation from others, due to the shame related to the behavior. They are commonly overweight, though may be normal weight. The diagnosis does not require an overconcern with shape or weight—a feature of both anorexia nervosa (AN) and BN—but this is nonetheless a frequent finding in individuals meeting criteria for BED and more common than that in overweight individuals without BED.

The female-to-male predominance in BED is less marked than has been found for AN and BN, with estimates showing a lifetime prevalence of BED in the USA of approximately 3 % in women and 2 % in men. The prevalence in weight loss programs and treatment settings may be as high as 30 %. These estimates may be falsely low, as the diagnosis is often missed. Lack of awareness of the disorder among both clinicians and the general population leads to inadequate screening in clinical settings and limited help-seeking among individuals experiencing the symptoms of BED. Shame about their eating behaviors—present almost without exception in those with BED—also deters some patients from reporting their symptoms, delaying diagnosis and treatment. For these and other reasons, it is estimated that only 25 % of those with symptoms of BED may seek help.

Research indicates that obesity predates the other symptoms of BED in most patients. BED appears to have a chronic course, with a longer duration of symptoms than has been found in AN and BN. This may in part be due to the fact that many patients experience a delay in their diagnosis or never come to clinical attention. The clinical presentation of BED may fluctuate over time in an individual, with periods of more or less active symptoms. Patients may also have a history of other feeding or eating disorders, such as AN or BN, or may progress from BED to one of these other disorders. Comorbid psychiatric disorders are common in those with BED,

including anxiety disorders, depressive disorders, posttraumatic stress disorder, and, less often, substance use disorders [see Chap. 11 for more discussion of comorbidity in BED].

Research suggests an interplay of genetic and environmental factors in the development of the disorder, with a combination of neurotransmitter dysregulation (including the opioid and monoamine systems), impairments in impulse control and reward sensitivity, family history, and life experiences contributing to the presentation of BED. Individuals who develop BED may have long-standing concerns about appearance and a history of receiving critical comments about appearance early in life, high levels of perceived stress, low social support, or a pattern of impaired support-seeking and self-care.

BED negatively impacts health, functioning, and emotional wellness. BED increases the likelihood of developing diabetes mellitus, cardiovascular disease and metabolic syndrome, joint and mobility issues, sleep apnea, and depression, and appears to be a stronger risk factor for such conditions than obesity alone. Identifying BED and engaging the individual in treatment are important for these reasons. Improved recognition can be accomplished through increased awareness and enhanced screening in primary care and general mental health treatment settings, as well as weight management programs. Clinicians can screen for symptoms of BED by asking about a patient's eating habits and significant changes in weight; binge-eating can be assessed through a question such as "do you sometimes feel like your eating is out of control, or like you can't stop it?" Following a positive response to a general screening question, further assessment of the quality and frequency of binge-eating episodes, and the psychological and physical experience of the binges, will help to confirm the diagnosis. It is important to keep in mind that individuals with BED commonly experience their behaviors as shameful, making it important to maintain a sensitive and non-judgmentally curious stance when exploring symptoms.

Once a diagnosis of BED is suspected or identified, a treatment plan can be developed to address the binge-eating episodes, comorbid psychiatric conditions and associated psychological and social difficulties, and any coexisting medical issues, including obesity. Most cases of BED can be treated in the ambulatory setting. A multimodal treatment approach ideally would include input

from mental health, primary care, and nutrition. Psychotherapy is the preferred first-line treatment for BED, with the most evidence for Cognitive Behavioral Therapy (CBT) and Interpersonal Therapy (IPT). CBT—which is usually offered individually or in a group, but which can also be accomplished through a self-help program (e.g., workbooks or online tools) if the patient is located in an area without access to in-person treatment—focuses on reducing the frequency of binge-eating episodes through behavioral interventions and addressing problematic thinking that perpetuates the cycle of binge-eating, low self-esteem, and limited coping skills. CBT has demonstrated good efficacy in BED, with abstinence from binge-eating in the majority of patients and sustained remission rates. IPT is an alternate first-line treatment for BED, with similar response rates as seen with CBT. In IPT for BED, the binge-eating symptoms are seen as a response to one of the core interpersonal problems of grief, role disputes, role transitions, or interpersonal deficits. The binge-eating symptoms are not addressed as directly as they are in CBT, and the treatment largely focuses on improving the person's interpersonal challenges, such as learning to prioritize self-care, advocate for one's needs, and utilize social supports. Other treatments have been studied in BED, including Dialectical Behavior Therapy, family therapy, and psychodynamic psychotherapy, but with less robust evidence for these modalities, CBT and IPT are preferred initial treatments.

Psychopharmacological management of BED can be useful in combination with psychotherapy and could be considered a reasonable option alone (though less effective than either CBT or IPT) in situations where the patient does not have access to psychotherapy. There is evidence for selective serotonin reuptake inhibitors (preferred first-line treatment based on expert recommendations due to their safety and tolerability profile), antiepileptic drugs (e.g., topiramate), and stimulant medications (e.g., lisdexamfetamine). Comorbid psychiatric conditions, such as depression or anxiety disorders, may benefit from psychopharmacologic management. Antiobesity medications are not specifically recommended because of the lack of evidence of efficacy in BED and the potential for serious adverse effects (e.g., cardiovascular events).

Behavioral weight loss programs can be considered in the approach to patients with BED. Nutritional counseling, goal-setting regarding food intake, encouragement of physical exercise, and

development of coping strategies to utilize in lieu of excessive calorie ingestion may improve some of the symptoms of BED; though binge-eating may not specifically be addressed, the effect may be to reduce the frequency and intensity of these episodes. Behavioral weight loss programs have not been found to be as effective as formal psychotherapy at achieving symptomatic improvement and remission in patients with BED, but could be considered in addition to psychotherapy for BED (or instead of psychotherapy in situations where the patient has limited access to such services).

Some patients may prefer self-help groups, one of the more well-known of which being Overeaters Anonymous (OA), a 12-step program modeled after Alcoholics Anonymous, developed for individuals with symptoms of eating disorders, including AN, BN, and BED. Similar to AA, OA meetings offer the opportunity to seek help on a drop-in basis through peer support and the structure of the 12-step program. OA emphasizes group fellowship, acknowledgment of the loss of control over binge-eating symptoms, and surrender to a higher power. "Abstinence" (from binge-eating and, in some cases, from certain "trigger foods") is a common principle discussed and practiced. As with AA, though on a smaller scale, OA meetings are available at no cost (with requests for contributions) in many areas across the USA and internationally. There are little published data on the efficacy of OA for individuals with eating disorders and no way to control the quality of help offered in any given meeting; however, for individuals for whom the 12-step model is appealing, or those without other effective treatment options available, engagement in OA could be reasonable to consider recommending.

General principles that can be useful when engaging and working with individuals with BED include encouraging flexible self-restraint with eating (overly rigid rules about eating may have the opposite of intended effect, causing more binge-eating due to the patient's sense of being unable to follow the rules perfectly or due to excessive deprivation), while addressing low self-esteem, self-criticism, and impaired body image; enhancing stress management skills; and encouraging more active engagement of one's social network and supports. Shame, stigma, and long-standing secrecy about their symptoms can be challenges in working with these individuals; a nonjudgmental approach, with

psychoeducation and instilling of hope, may enhance the patient's ability to connect and engage in treatment.

Overall, treatment for BED can be quite effective, with CBT demonstrating sustained remission rates in up to 70 % of patients. Bariatric surgery, though not specifically a treatment for BED, is not contraindicated in patients with BED and may assist with weight loss in obese individuals whether or not they have BED. Careful screening prior to bariatric surgery, however, is essential, as patients who continue to binge-eat after surgery have worse outcome than those who abstain from binge-eating. Evaluating readiness to adapt to a new way of eating, with small meals and absence of binge-eating, as well as reviewing the overall tendency toward poor impulse control and general coping skills when under stress, may help the clinician to identify those patients who are more appropriate for this surgical intervention and those for whom the risks may outweigh the benefits.

9.3   Differential Diagnosis

Most commonly, the presenting signs and symptoms of Binge Eating Disorder will appear to overlap with those of bulimia nervosa, obesity, and anorexia nervosa. Patients in any of these categories may binge-eat. Patients with AN are significantly underweight, with persistent behavior to prevent weight gain, making it usually more easily distinguishable from BED, where repeated behavior to lose weight is not a primary feature of the disorder, and in which patients are most often, but not always, overweight.

Individuals who are obese or overweight may frequently overeat and may engage in binge-eating, but what is less pronounced in these individuals is the negative experience of the binge episode, as well as the degree of distress related to the eating patterns. Such individuals, in the absence of these pathological findings, do not have an eating disorder. Compared to individuals who are overweight, with or without binge-eating behavior, patients with BED are more likely to have negative health outcomes, including the overall poorer physical health, worse metabolic profiles (such as lipid and glucose regulation), more unhealthy patterns of weight

gain (frequently more rapid), and poorer response to weight loss treatments. Not included in the diagnostic criteria for BED, but a common finding nonetheless, individuals with BED are also more likely than their overweight counterparts without BED to have a negative experience of their bodies, including more pronounced concern with shape and weight.

BED can be distinguished from BN by the presence or absence of recurrent compensatory behavior to "undo" calorie intake; in BN, these behaviors are a prominent component of the disorder, whereas in BED, if they are present, they are rare and not a core focus of attention.

As with BN, the clinician can also consider in the differential diagnosis of BED those medical disorders involving hyperphagia, such as Prader–Willi syndrome and Kleine–Levin syndrome. These conditions, however, are not associated with the psychological symptoms of BED, including the negative emotional experiences associated with the binge episodes in BED. Some medications, such as sedative–hypnotic medications taken for sleep, have been linked to binge-eating without memory of the event the next day, and this could be considered in the evaluation of a patient with binge-eating behavior who is taking sleeping medications, such as zolpidem.

9.4   Outcome

Ian engaged quickly with Dr. Jarvis, explaining that he feels so "fed up" with his eating, and how it seems to be influencing his family life, his mood, and his physical health, that he wants to "get this fixed." He was able to talk quite openly about how the binge episodes seem to be "triggered" as a way to soothe negative feelings, such as stress about his work or relationships; there is an initial relief, which is quickly followed by remorse for the eating, then feeling worse about himself, and creating a vicious cycle that seems to lead to even more binge-eating, decrease in self-esteem, and weight gain. He is sure his wife knows about his episodes but does not feel he can speak to her about them due to the shame he feels about them. Ian did not fulfill the criteria for a depressive disorder or an anxiety disorder and denied substance use issues.

Dr. Jarvis facilitated Ian's referral to an eating disorder program where he began a course of CBT for BED. He was also referred to a nutritionist. After several sessions with the nutritionist and therapy, Ian felt ready to involve his wife in his treatment. He decided that he would benefit from starting Weight Watchers—"I could use the extra social reinforcement to lose some of this weight!", and his wife, who also wanted to lose a few pounds, went to his first meeting with him. Dr. Jarvis did not feel that medications were needed, and Ian preferred to avoid them, as well. Over the next six moths, Ian lost 25 lb and was exercising more and generally being more physically active on weekends, enjoying playing outside with his children and taking walks with the whole family. He felt a new sense of confidence and less stress related to his work and family. He was able to stop binge-eating; when he had impulses to do so, he would take a walk or talk to his wife. He reported to Dr. Jarvis that he occasionally ate "more than I should —I've never been the poster child for self-control, doc!", but he no longer felt out of control of his eating and was able to shrug off these indulgences without negative emotional consequences.

Suggested Readings

Citrome L. A primer on binge eating disorder diagnosis and management. CNS spectr. 2015;20(S1):41–51.

Kessler RM, Hutson PH, Herman BK, Potenza MN. The neurobiological basis of binge-eating disorder. Neurosci Biobehav Rev. 2016;63:223–38.

McElroy SL, Guerdjikova AI, Mori N, Munos MR, Keck PE. Overview of the treatment of binge eating disorder. CNS Spectr. 2015;20:546–56.

Vocks S, Tuschen-Caffier B, Pietrowsky R, Rustenbach SJ, Kersting A, Herpertz S. Meta-analysis of the effectiveness of psychological and pharmacological treatments for binge eating disorder. Int J Eat Disord. 2010;43:205–17.

Chapter 10
James, the Inconsistent Eater

10.1 Case Presentation

James is 31-year-old man, a former high school wrestler and now a participant in endurance sports, who is seeing Dr. Kerr for the first time at the prompting of his internist because of concerns for an eating disorder. James tells Dr. Kerr that he is sure he does not have an eating disorder, but that he would be grateful if Dr. Kerr had any suggestions for books he could read about controlling his food intake. James goes on to report that he was a successful varsity wrestler in high school, competing in a weight class at least 15 lb lighter than he felt his body would naturally have been. He maintained his weight during wrestling season (115 lb, height 5'7"; BMI 18) by drastically cutting calories before meets, and other techniques widely used by others on the team, such as forced sweating through working out in hot conditions/heavy clothing, diuretic use, and occasionally self-induced vomiting if he had eaten too much or after having a few beers ("that's a lot of calories!") at a party.

After an injury halted his wrestling career in college, he relaxed his eating and exercise, and his weight slowly crept up over the next five years to 180 lbs. In his mid-20s, frustrated with the extra weight he was carrying and unsatisfied in his work and personal

© Springer International Publishing Switzerland 2017 95
J. Gordon-Elliott, *Fundamentals of Diagnosing and Treating Eating Disorders*, DOI 10.1007/978-3-319-46065-9_10

life, he began cycling with a friend from work ("a total endurance junkie"). He increased his cycling to 100-mile rides and then began running and swimming with the hopes of doing triathlons. He has competed in a "half Ironman triathalon" (1.2-mile swim, 56-mile bike ride, and 13.1-mile run) and plans to begin training for a full Ironman soon.

He reads a lot about diet and optimizing his "racing weight" and thinks that at his current weight of 150 lb he is probably about 7–10 lb above this "ideal" weight that would enhance his performance. He is frustrated that he cannot seem to drop his weight lower, despite the number of miles he cycles, runs, and swims every week. He describes a diet that is relatively low in carbohydrates and high in protein and (mostly) healthy fats. With some prompting, he admits that one or two times a week he will get "so hungry" that he will eat a lot of starchy food late at night, such as 2 bags of chips or a large pizza.

Occasionally he will self-induce vomiting after these episodes, explaining that he is concerned about how the ingested food and water weight will affect his next workout. He will try to restrict his food intake more the next day but admits that sometimes this makes him more likely to overeat again. He drinks minimal alcohol. He denies feeling "fat," but he says he will look at himself in the mirror some days for 10 or 15 min, inspecting every angle and chastising himself for areas that do not look toned enough or telling himself that he does not look "like an athlete."

10.2   Diagnosis/Assessment

Preferred diagnosis: No diagnosis.

10.3   Differential Diagnosis

James is a man who most likely does not have a diagnosable eating disorder; however, he engages in disordered eating that could put him at risk, physically and emotionally, and thus could benefit from clinical attention.

James's story is a fairly common one—a former competitive athlete who stops competing due to injury, a change in priorities, or awareness of limitations of his potential, who then reengages in sport later in life with all the drive of his former athletic self. In the intervening years, the individual's intense and somewhat compulsive nature may be gratified in other ways, such as through long hours at work or aggressive engagement in recreational activities (parties, heavy drinking, drug use, etc.). In the context of rediscovering an athletic focus of attention, the person may redirect much of that energy back into physical achievement, becoming increasingly focused on performance enhancement, which—in sports—means a focus on the body. In endurance sports (as discussed in Chap. 5), performance can be directly correlated with a lean and light body composition. The competitive endurance athlete will therefore aim to optimize lean body mass and minimize unnecessary weight. This will ideally be accomplished through an optimal balance of "calories in" and "calories out," involving the burning of calories during training and monitoring food intake. Extra measures may be taken by the athlete if his or her weight remains higher than what he or she believes would be best for performance; this might include further reduction of calorie intake or burning excess calories through additional exercise beyond the normal training routine. This is where the athlete may begin to walk (or, perhaps, more aptly stated, "run") the fine line between weight loss for performance enhancement and the development of a pattern of disordered eating and exercise. Preoccupation with weight loss or weight maintenance may lead to more aberrant behaviors, such as self-induced vomiting, or laxative or diuretic misuse. The individual may also become more fixated on body image. The focus on numbers on the scale or inches on the measuring tape, which originally had been a means to the end of increased performance, may get distorted over time, becoming the goal, itself.

The endurance athlete who wants to be competitive will likely need to experience some degree of deprivation—avoidance of certain foods or drinks that would add weight or otherwise impair performance. This athlete might weigh himself daily and cut back on calories further if the number on the scale goes higher. Within this population, such behavior would be within the range of "normal." At what point, then, would it be appropriate to consider

diagnosing a feeding and eating disorder, or attempting to engage the athlete in treatment? Is there a cutoff or certain behaviors that would indicate that the patient has slipped into the "pathologic" range?

James is not underweight and is not engaging in ways to obstruct maintaining a healthy weight, and therefore does not have anorexia nervosa (AN). He is vomiting as a compensatory mechanism, and his body image may be having an undue influence on his self-esteem, raising the possibility of bulimia nervosa (BN). He is vomiting less frequently than once a week; one could consider his restriction after a binge, or any increase in exercise that he engages in after a binge, as compensatory behaviors. However, with further questioning, he admits that the post-binge restriction usually only involves reduction of approximately 100 calories the next day, and that he rarely substantially increases his exercise after a binge to "make up" for it. He eats excessively at least once a week in a way that he experiences as a binge (with a sense of loss of control and resultant guilt/regret), and therefore, he would technically fulfill criteria for binge eating disorder (BED). The value of diagnosing BED in this case could be questioned; further elaboration will be discussed below.

Eating disorders in general, as touched upon in Chap. 5, are more common in competitive athletes than in the general population. Higher rates of AN and BN have been found in elite athletes [1, 2, 4]; more common than either of these, however, are sub-syndromal or mixed symptomatology disorders, such as occasional use of compensatory mechanisms to remove calories that does not meet the frequency criteria of BN, or excessive calorie restriction and refusal to gain weight but without the reported body image distortions of AN [3]. Though most of these individuals might not receive a formal diagnosis of an eating disorder, that does not mean that they are not at risk; in fact, patterns of disordered eating will increase the chances of developing a full-criteria eating disorder in the future, and—even if not meeting criteria for a diagnosable disorder—the eating- and food-related behaviors may still put the individual at risk for physical and emotional complications.

As was alluded to earlier, diagnosis of an eating disorder may be more complicated in the setting of a competitive athlete who, in the "normal" pursuit in high-level achievement, may manipulate his or her diet, or be more focused on weight and inches, in ways that a

non-athlete might not. The diagnoses of AN and BN include some assessment of the extent to which the individual's body image is a focal point of attention. In athletes, specifically, there may be substantial preoccupation with body weight and composition but the athlete might fully deny any distortion of his or her body image or any psychological consequences of the body focus—rather, the athlete may explain that the body needs to be in the optimal state in order to perform best. In situations where disordered behavior around food and weight reduction begins leading to impaired achievement (such as when the individual becomes very low weight, and lean muscle mass is substantially reduced and performance suffers), it can be more straightforward to assess for distorted body image—the patient may continue to state that these manipulations of the body are needed for performance despite incontrovertible evidence disproving that. But in most cases, this is less clear; the athlete (and coach, nutritionist, even physician) will not necessarily have a sense of the physical parameters and food intake profile that will best serve the athlete's performance. In such cases, it may take more time, observation, and exploration with the patient about how his or her behaviors are affecting other areas of physical, social, and emotional functioning, to determine the extent to which body image and ideas about weight and diet have become distorted.

How can Dr. Kerr approach James in a way that is most likely to engage him and help him? There is no right answer, but—as a general principle in patient-care—an individual will more readily collaborate in treatment if there is a vested interest in a benefit the treatment might provide. Aggressive confrontation with James about his having an eating disorder (which, he has already emphatically stated at the outset of the first appointment with Dr. Kerr, he does *not* have) may distance him further. On the other hand, engaging him as an athlete, validating his efforts to be as competitive and successful as he can be, could be a good start. The simple act of pointing out that the binges seem to occur in the context of calorie deficit (triggering extra intake to compensate for the deficit, and usually overcompensating) might catch his interest and offer him hope that there might be a solution (e.g., changing his eating schedule to minimize the extreme hunger leading to a binge). Using the word "bulimia" might further alienate James, but talking with him about the negative physical impact of vomiting

(electrolyte disturbance, tooth enamel erosion, gastrointestinal problems, etc. [see Chap. 7 for further discussion of BN]) could be a useful approach. One could argue that it might not even be helpful or appropriate to assign the diagnosis of binge eating disorder to James, as his binges appear to be occurring in response to a calorie deficit, and nutritional counseling as well as psychoeducation about stress-management may in fact help him undo this pattern of eating behavior.

The clinician should be honest and straightforward. Binge-eating and self-induced vomiting are unhealthy behaviors that can escalate and lead to substantial negative physical and emotional outcomes; this should be expressed to the patient. Communicating this in a way that is clear but compassionate is more challenging, but this is the art of clinical care. Understanding a patient and his or her personality, goals, expectations, and values will allow the provider to present information in a way that is acceptable and meaningful to the patient, planting the seeds of engagement and eventual change.

10.4 Outcome

Gauging appropriately that James prefers to think in pragmatic terms, with logical connections and not a lot of "fluff," and also appreciating that James is very competitive, Dr. Kerr engaged James's issues as a problem to "solve" together. He validated James's competitive nature by expressing that he shared the goal of helping James perform as best as possible. He likened James's body to a "machine" that needed to be fueled and also maintained. Without pulling punches, he told James that purging could be dangerous and would be the most important thing to stop immediately; however, he added that they would do what they can to help James do this without feeling like he is losing control of his weight goals. He went on to add that perhaps some of the things that James is doing to feel "in control" are actually leading him to feel even more out of control (and to engage in unhealthy and frankly unsafe behaviors). James was struck by this idea and

curious to learn more about why that might be happening. Dr. Kerr gave James a referral to a sports nutritionist and also suggested that James begin working with a coach rather than determining his training plan on his own. He also suggested that they begin a course of psychotherapy—with the goal of understanding some aspects of the way James's mind works to see if they might help him optimize his athletic potential. Interestingly, but not surprisingly, this led to a very fruitful course of psychotherapy, in which James was able to process many lifelong emotional issues that had been causing him difficulties in his work and relationships. His binge-eating slowly disappeared and he maintained a healthy weight while successfully competing in many endurance events.

References

1. Chatterton JM, Petrie TA. Prevalence of disordered eating and pathogenic weight control behaviors among male collegiate athletes. Eat Disord. 2013;21(4):328–41.
2. Hulley AJ, Hill AJ. Eating disorders and health in elite women distance runners. Int J Eat Disord. 2001;30(3):312–7.
3. Petrie TA, Rogers R. Extending the discussion of eating disorders to include men and athletes. J Couns Psychol. 2001;29:743–53.
4. Sundgot-Borgen J, Torstveit MK. Prevalence of eating disorders in elite athletes is higher than in the general population. Clin J Sport Med. 2004;14 (1):25–32.

Suggested Reading

Goltz FR, Stenzel LM, Schneider CD. Disordered eating behaviors and body image in male athletes. Rev Braz Psiquiatr. 2013;35(3):237–42.

Chapter 11
Kendra's Social Anxiety

11.1 Case Presentation

Kendra is a 28-year-old former US Army nurse, honorably discharged after 17 months of active duty in Afghanistan following a knee injury requiring surgery and extensive rehabilitation, who is coming for her first appointment with Dr. Levine, a primary care doctor in an ambulatory care clinic. Kendra reports having a history of migraines, but otherwise is not aware of any major medical problems. She admits that it has been 2 years since she is come to see a physician: "I'm embarrassed to say it, but I haven't been taking great care of myself." She admits that while she was very active before and during her military days, after returning home from the service and completing her allotted six weeks of physical therapy sessions, she stopped exercising and started eating more "junk". She does not know how much weight she has gained, but says she has started to wear oversized clothes without dress sizes because "I don't really want to know my size." She says she is uncomfortable with how she looks. She states that she lives near her parents and her older sister (who is married with children) and reports not having many other friends. She describes feeling acutely nervous when she imagines meeting new people or socializing in group settings, saying that she is uncomfortable with

how she looks: "I've always been terrible at small talk—I just can't do it and I freeze up." She says that recently being around people other than her family has made her "want to go home and eat a bag of cookies," but then she trails off and does not finish her thought.

Kendra reports that her knee injury was sustained while working in the field, attempting to recover and save a soldier who was wounded near a bomb-making compound. A comrade there with her detonated a mine while they were approaching the wounded soldier, and Kendra fell to her side after the explosion, twisting her knee and tearing her anterior cruciate ligament. She could not get up and saw her comrade unconscious and bleeding near her, unable to act and not knowing what to do. She then says to Dr. Levine that she would prefer to stop talking about the event as it is "easier for me to put stuff like that away."

While writing his note later in the day, Dr. Levine had more questions about Kendra, and listed those he wanted to address in their next visit. He was curious to hear more about her eating habits, wondering what she meant about eating the cookies (was she describing binge-eating behavior?), as well as about her anxiety in social settings and the emotional consequences of her experiences in the military, including the day she was injured. He spoke to a psychiatrist colleague in the ambulatory care center, who also wondered whether Kendra might have a history of traumatic events other than the day of her injury, based on her comment about "putting stuff like that away"—had there been other experiences in her life "like that"?

11.2 Diagnosis/Assessment

Kendra fulfills diagnostic criteria for social anxiety disorder (SAD) and perhaps generalized anxiety disorder (GAD). Dr. Levine strongly suspects an eating disorder, specifically binge eating disorder (BED). He also wonders about trauma and an additional diagnosis of posttraumatic stress disorder (PTSD).

Kendra's presentation is typical for patients with BED [see Chap. 9 for further discussion of BED]. It may be more common than not for an individual with BED to have another co-occurring mental illness, with studies showing that two-thirds have received

an anxiety disorder diagnosis, almost one-half have been diagnosed with a depressive or bipolar disorder, and nearly one-quarter have fulfilled criteria for a substance use disorder. Personality disorders are equally common, occurring in nearly one-third of patients diagnosed with BED; avoidant personality disorder is a particularly common one, which shares many features of anxiety disorders, notably SAD [1]. In fact, it is most often the other mental disorders that bring these patients to clinical attention, not the eating symptoms. As discussed in Chap. 9, lack of awareness about BED as a validated and treatable condition, as well as shame regarding eating symptoms, may limit help-seeking in individuals with binge-eating behaviors and full-syndrome BED. Even when they come to attention, they may preferentially discuss other symptoms, such as depressive or anxiety symptoms, for all of the same reasons. Clinicians, too, may not think to screen for disordered eating symptoms or—even if they suspect them—may not know how to ask. Recognizing that binge eating behavior may accompany various other psychiatric conditions may help to prompt the clinician to begin asking patients about their eating behaviors and may help to detect cases of BED and other feeding and eating disorders that would have remained undiagnosed. Detection, in turn, will open up the possibility for treatment.

It has been suggested that for most patients with eating disorders and another psychiatric disorder, the onset of the eating disorder occurred after the development of other psychiatric symptoms, indicating that—at least for some—eating disorder symptoms may manifest in a susceptible individual in the setting of particular mental health states (e.g., Major Depression). Individuals who respond to stress by developing anxiety and depressive symptoms may be particularly prone to binge eating behavior. Theoretically, these may be people who are more likely to experience themselves negatively and to be reluctant to engage others as emotional supports and resources, turning inwards to cope with their distress. Binge eating, which will elicit immediate gratification through triggering a neurobiological reward response, may become a coping strategy the person turns to over and over—with time, developing into a habit-based behavior. This, in turn, becomes a vicious cycle, as the binge eating (and the commonly associated weight gain) becomes something the person is ashamed of, leading to additional impairment of self-esteem and social withdrawal.

PTSD may be particularly linked to BED, perhaps through shared environmental and psychological risk factors. Studies show that female military personnel (a rapidly growing group over recent years) may have relatively high rates of co-occurrence of PTSD and BED. Indeed the literature appears to support that lifetime exposure to trauma may increase an individual's risk for developing binge-eating symptoms and BED, hypothetically with binge-eating resulting as a mechanism for coping with distressing emotional experiences. It has been shown that individuals with a history of adverse childhood experiences, especially emotional abuse, are more likely to engage in emotional eating (eating in response to emotional dysregulation, ostensibly in an effort to better modulate the distress) and appear to be more likely to develop eating disorder pathology in adulthood. Individuals with frank trauma-related symptoms (e.g., re-experiencing, hypervigilance, and negative mood) may engage in binge-eating to manage these specific symptoms; for example, insomnia related to hypervigilance or nightmares may trigger binge-eating at night to help soothe distress or allow the patient to fall asleep. Shame, which, as mentioned, is commonly related to binge-eating behavior, may also be present in individuals with symptoms of PTSD—perhaps due to their sense that they should be able to "get over" the trauma or because the trauma-related symptoms reveal some weakness of character. Such shame may make it even less likely for a person experiencing PTSD and binge-eating symptoms to ask for help (from loved ones or health care professionals) or disclose their symptoms without prompting.

11.2.1   Management

Given how common it can be for a patient to present with symptoms of more than one psychiatric condition, the evaluation can be very challenging for the provider who is trying to not only establish diagnoses, but also prioritize the list of problems and develop an optimal treatment plan [see Chap. 8 for further discussion of the approach to the differential diagnosis]. There are various ways to approach this clinical task. One can choose to review criteria for as many conditions as possible (time permitting!) and assign every

diagnosis for which criteria have been met. This approach is thorough but can be onerous and perhaps lead to the problem of overdiagnosing. Alternatively, the clinician may choose to view some symptoms as secondary to one diagnosis, rather than a separate disorder. This may allow for a more concise problem list, though may not always be appropriate or feasible, and may lead to not addressing a disorder that is present and treatable.

In the case of Kendra, her binge eating symptoms might be viewed as a symptom of her SAD (as a way of coping with her anxiety), and the clinician might choose to actively treat the anxiety disorder (perhaps with a combination of an antidepressant and cognitive behavioral therapy targeting her distorted thoughts related to social interactions), expecting the binge symptoms to improve as the SAD remits. In many cases, this might be the most appropriate strategy. On the other hand, one could argue that by considering the eating symptoms as a symptom of the anxiety disorder, Kendra may be lose the opportunity to receive specific and effective treatments for her binge eating. In addition, it may be challenging to determine which disorder is "primary" and which symptoms are "secondary". In the case of Kendra, does she binge eat to cope with her social anxiety, or is she socially avoidant because of her binge eating and related shame, or some combination of both?

As is true throughout clinical medicine, real world scenarios are never as clean as the books and diagnoses would have us believe, and algorithms and diagnostic criteria will only get us so far. Arguably, the best we can do is to be as aware as possible of typical scenarios and common comorbidities, and to be sensitive to cues that the patient is offering. In the case of Kendra, perhaps the wisest approach would involve teasing out her various symptoms (including social anxiety, trauma-related, and eating symptoms); determining as best as possible which symptoms are more urgently in need of attention, or which might be more quickly treatable; and then establishing a treatment plan, with ongoing modification as needed. Accepting our own limitations, and being open to reassessing a situation and changing our formulation and treatment plan when new information is available, are essential ingredients of good clinical care, without which we may fail to offer the patient the most comprehensive and compassionate care.

11.3 Differential Diagnosis

As reviewed above, symptoms of BED may be comorbid with, or may present as a feature of, other diagnoses, including depressive and bipolar disorders, anxiety disorders, trauma-related disorders, substance use disorders, and personality disorders, as well as other eating disorders. In the case of Kendra, a woman with a trauma history, social avoidance, binge-eating, and weight gain, it would be important to fully review criteria for SAD, PTSD, BED, as well as major depressive disorder and GAD. As substance use disorders can masquerade as nearly any other disorder, and because they can so frequently coexist with anxiety and trauma-related disorders, it will be important to rule out any substance use issues—especially as, in this case, they could be contributing to social withdrawal, weight gain (e.g., if she is drinking excessive alcohol), and binge-eating in an impulsive, intoxicated state. Dissociative disorders might also be considered, as binge-eating may occur in the setting of a dissociative state, which a patient like Kendra might be more prone to given her history of trauma and a possible trauma-related disorder.

11.4 Outcome

Over the course of her next two visits with Kendra, Dr. Levine was able to collect more meaningful history. Kendra disclosed binge-eating happening twice a week—a symptom that she had occasionally engaged in as a teenager but which had become more frequent in the setting of her recent stressors. She also screened positive for some trauma-related symptoms but did not meet full criteria for PTSD. She wanted help with her social anxiety symptoms but felt unable to break the negative cycle she was in of binge-eating, then feeling worse about herself the next day, further social avoidance, and then further binge-eating. Dr. Levine chose to begin structured treatment for BED, as this appeared to be the symptom that Kendra was most troubled by and most motivated to change; in addition, it seemed that without addressing this symptom, it would be challenging to make progress with her social

anxiety and other symptoms. The treatment plan included psychoeducation, nutritional counseling, and engagement in behavior modification [see Chap. 9 for further discussion]. Over time, Kendra's binge-eating subsided. The work she was doing on her eating made her feel proud of herself and more confident in what she could accomplish. She began getting more exercise, allowing her to participate more actively in physical therapy, with further improvement in her mobility and pain. She gradually became more social, making a friend at the physical therapy gym, and getting involved in activities at her local Veterans' Affairs health care center. With time, she was able to talk more with Dr. Levine about her response to her experiences in the military. She disclosed a history of trauma as a child and began to explore how this had shaped her subsequent experiences. Her mood improved and she felt satisfied with her life in ways she had not for many years.

Reference

1. Hudson JI, Hiripi E, Pope HG, Kessler RC. The prevalence and correlates of eating disorders in the national comorbidity survey replication. Biol Psychiatry. 2007;61:348–58.

Suggested Readings

Burns EE, Fischer S, Jackson JL, Harding HG. Deficits in emotion regulation mediate the relationship between childhood abuse and later eating disorder symptoms. Child Abuse Negl. 2012;36:32–9.

Kong S, Bernstein K. Childhood trauma as a predictor of eating psychopathology and its mediating variables in patients with eating disorders. J Clin Nurs. 2009;18:1897–907.

Michopoulos V, Powers A, Moore C, Villarreal S, Ressler KJ, Bradley B. The mediating role of emotion dysregulation and depression on the relationship between childhood trauma exposure and emotional eating. Appetite. 2015;91:129–36.

Rosenbaum DL, Kimerling R, Pomernacki A, Goldstein KM, Yano EM, Sadler AG, Carney D, Bastian LA, Bean-Mayberry BA, Frayne SM. Binge eating among women veterans in primary care: comborbidities and treatment priorities. Women's Health Issues. 2016; [Epub ahead of print].

Chapter 12
Lisa, Overweight but Undernourished

12.1 Case Presentation

Lisa is a 32-year-old woman, mother of 3 children, prescribed citalopram by her primary care provider for a diagnosis of generalized anxiety disorder (GAD), who is referred to the nurse practitioner in her medical clinic, Mr. Norman, for help with weight loss. Lisa came to see her primary physician, Dr. Munn, for the first time in 3 years. Her weight, which had been 155 lb before her third pregnancy, is now 180 lb one year after the baby was born. At 5′3″, her body mass index (BMI) is 32. Lisa admits to Mr. Norman that she has had a hard time "losing the baby weight." She describes eating many of the same foods her children eat ("it is what I have around!"), including macaroni and cheese and chicken nuggets. She is not sure what she could do to improve her diet. When asked about exercise, she says she's "never been much of an exerciser" and also does not think she would be able to find time to do any. She lives in a small suburban community; the local gym is 30 min away in the next town. Elaborating on her history, she explains she has been "a little heavy" since adolescence, though she has progressively gained more weight that she has not been able to lose with each pregnancy. When asked about her emotional health, she explains that she tends to be "a worrier" and gets very anxious if she does not hear from her

© Springer International Publishing Switzerland 2017   111
J. Gordon-Elliott, *Fundamentals of Diagnosing and Treating
Eating Disorders*, DOI 10.1007/978-3-319-46065-9_12

husband at least twice a day ("I know it is silly, but I worry
something has happened to him—like a car accident or something!"). She describes frequent headaches and some difficulty
sleeping when she is particularly stressed. She admits that she will
turn to food sometimes when she feels a lot of anxiety, for example,
going to the local fast food restaurant to pick up 2 burgers on her
way to pick up her oldest child from school. Occasionally, when she
cannot sleep, she will eat "a whole lot" of food (e.g., a box of the
kids' cereal, and half a box of cookies). This happens once or twice
a month. She feels upset about it the next morning. She denies
restricting calories or any efforts to compensate for her eating, such
as vomiting or laxative use. She expresses a desire to lose "a few
pounds," but adds "I wouldn't even know where to start!"

12.2   Diagnosis/Assessment

Preferred Diagnosis: Generalized Anxiety Disorder
    Lisa is overweight but does not fulfill criteria for a feeding and
eating disorder. With a BMI of 32, she is in the obese range [see
Text Box: body mass index (BMI) for calculation and ranges]. She
has gained excess weight in the past five years, going from the
"overweight" range to the "obese" range. She occasionally eats
more than would be considered a "usual" amount and regrets her
intake, but this is not happening with the frequency or psychological features that would meet criteria for binge eating
disorder (BED). She has concerns about her weight and a decline
in self-confidence related to her body image, but does not engage
in restriction of food or other inappropriate compensatory behaviors to lose weight. [See Chap. 3 for more discussion of clinical
scenarios where weight, food, and body image are prominent
without meeting criteria for a feeding and eating disorder].

Body Mass Index (BMI)
BMI is computed by the following formula: body weight (in kilograms) divided by height squared (in centimeters).

BMI calculators and tables can be found online. See The National Institutes of Health:
http://www.nhlbi.nih.gov/health/educational/lose_wt/BMI/bmicalc.htm

BMI ranges:
Underweight = <18.5
Normal weight = 18.5–24.9
Overweight = 25–29.9
Obesity = 30 or greater

With a few exceptions, weight gain occurs when there is an overall calorie surplus—essentially, ingesting more calories a day than the body is burning. This will happen when an individual begins eating more calories, or when calorie expenditure drops. Increased calorie intake is a purely behavioral issue—the person is either eating more food or eating higher density food (e.g., food with a higher percent of fat, which has double the calories per gram than the other macronutrients: carbohydrates and protein). Many things can cause a person to eat more calories, including, but not limited to, a change in available food choices (e.g., switching from one workplace where healthy food options were available for lunch to a new workplace with a cafeteria where mostly high-fat foods are served); interpersonal factors (e.g., beginning a new relationship where many activities involve going out to restaurants for meals and possibly ingesting more alcohol than usual); increased hunger or perceived hunger (e.g., due to a new medication); or other psychological factors (e.g., elevated stress due to work or social issues, leading to "stress-eating" or "emotional eating"). It is worth noting that even an increase in exercise—something that would be considered a positive change and potentially associated with weight loss—can lead some individuals to gain weight; a modest boost in calorie expenditure may lead to a compensatory increase in hunger, with the effect that the individual begins eating more additional calories than the extra exercise is burning.

Whatever the reason a person has begun eating more calories, if this is not balanced with an increase in calorie burning, the net effect will be weight gain. This process may be something the individual is conscious of, or something that will happen gradually and seemingly "mindlessly," only to be noticed when the individual's clothes no longer fit the same, or when he or she gets on the scale for the first time in a while and notices a difference. It has been estimated that the gain or loss of one pound of weight is equivalent to approximately 3500 kilocalories (kcal, commonly known as "calories"). An increase of even 200 kcal per day (e.g., the amount found in a typical can of soda) will lead to a calorie excess of 6000 kcal per month, with a weight gain of 20 lb over a single year.

Of note, various psychotropic medications have been associated with weight gain, some more substantial than others. There is a clear association between certain antipsychotic medications (e.g., olanzapine and clozapine) and weight gain, and this may be primarily due to increased appetite via histamine receptor modulation and perhaps also reduced activity. The evidence is less clear for antidepressants, though there may be indication of modest weight gain from chronic use of selective serotonin reuptake inhibitors in some individuals. A review of the weight and metabolic effects of all psychotropic medications and medications given for other medical indications is beyond the scope of this book.

Decreased calorie expenditure may be related to behavior or physiologic factors. A person may burn fewer calories due to less physical activity (e.g., moving to a city where one drives more than walks, or because of an injury that limits physical activity). Physical and medical changes may affect calorie burning. For instance, reduction in muscle mass, due to aging or inactivity, will lead to a lower percent of lean body mass and a reduction of a person's basal metabolic rate (which is largely a function of the person's age, gender, and body composition). Medical conditions, such as hypothyroidism, may lower metabolic rate. A history of obesity will also impact calorie burning; it has been found that individuals who were previously obese may have a significantly lower basal metabolic rate than would be expected for their age, gender, weight, and body composition; this seems to be a result of homeostatic variables that are altered, perhaps irrevocably, in the obese state. Certain medications (e.g., olanzapine) have been

postulated to directly alter metabolic rate, independent of their effects on increasing appetite; the evidence remains unclear, though it is possible that certain medications may contribute to weight gain via a reduction in basal metabolic rate, perhaps through changes in body composition or endocrine changes.

Other factors may lead to weight gain that are not as closely linked to a net positive calorie balance (calories in > calories out). Increase in total body water will increase the individual's weight; this could be due to medical issues, such as heart failure or liver disease, or medications, such as lithium. A significant increase in muscle mass, due to heavy lifting, may result in an overall increase in weight despite a decrease in physical measurements, such as waist circumference and dress size; this is because of muscle's greater density than fat tissue.

Overweight and obesity have become a major public health issue in recent times. According to the World Health Organization (WHO), the prevalence of obesity has doubled worldwide since 1980. Records from 2014 found that nearly 40 % of the world's adult population was overweight, and 13 % were in the obese range; rates are higher in the USA. Obesity in childhood has also increased over the past 40 years [3]. Numerous factors, from changes in the way food is prepared and made available, to alterations in time spent being physically active, to disturbances in regulation of weight and other metabolic factors (perhaps through increased exposure to chemicals through food and the environment), all seem to have coalesced, with the result of higher rates of weight-related issues— interestingly (and most likely not coincidentally) at a time when eating disorders and focus on body image in the media have become increasingly pervasive. The food industry has made food progressively more "fast"—highly palatable, pre-processed food containing enhanced levels of fat, sugar, and flavor additives that excessively stimulate the senses, taking advantage of natural reward signals related to food (a requirement for survival), and leading to excessive intake of fast, cheap food with immediate pleasurable effects, and long-lasting negative effects (expanding waistlines, rising rates of diabetes, dyslipidemia, and end-organ disease) [2]. At the same time, images of nearly impossible to achieve standards of thinness saturate the media. The cognitive and emotional dissonance caused by these conflicting trends create (idealization of thinness despite a heavier population) can be confusing, to say the

least; for susceptible individuals, the psychological effects of these mixed messages can be frankly psychologically destructive and may contribute to the development of feeding and eating disorders, from anorexia nervosa to BED.

The impact of excess weight on physical and mental health is substantial and complex. Medical consequences of obesity may relate to the metabolic syndrome that will often accompany obesity, increasing an individual's risk for cardiovascular and cerebrovascular disease, diabetes, and dementia. Excess fat may also be associated with osteoarthritis, chronic pain, chronic inflammation, and cancer. Obesity may contribute to the development or perpetuation of mental health issues, such as anxiety and depression, perhaps through a combination of psychological factors (e.g., low self-esteem, interpersonal stressors) and neurobiological mechanisms related to obesity (e.g., systemic inflammation or disruption of the endocrine system). Elevated risk for some of the more significant medical consequences of obesity appears to be related to certain metabolic factors; individuals with a larger waist circumference (greater than 40 inches for men, greater than 35 inches for women) have more visceral fat, which is associated with higher rates of diabetes, hypercholesterolemia, and general inflammation.

On the other hand, it is possible to be relatively healthy and overweight. An individual, for example, who is in the obese range of BMI, but carries most of her weight in her hips and lower body, as opposed to her midsection, and who has normal lipid profiles and a normal fasting glucose, may potentially have the same cardiovascular risk factors as an individual with a BMI in the normal range. For this reason and others, it is important to keep in mind that measures such as the BMI or an isolated total cholesterol level can be useful but may be misleading; the entire picture—including the various biophysical parameters and less tangible factors such as quality of life and satisfaction with one's body—should be assessed as a whole.

12.2.1 Management

For the vast majority of cases of weight gain leading to overweight and obesity, the problem is behavioral—too many calories in and too few calories out. Doing a thorough screening of Lisa's eating

habits, exercise patterns, and approach to eating and physical activity would be useful. She would benefit from a comprehensive assessment by her primary care doctor for the evaluation of medical issues or medications that could be contributing, as well as modifiable health risk factors, such as dyslipidemia, hypertension, and diabetes. A full psychiatric history should also be done to identify any psychiatric diagnoses that may be contributing to the weight issues—including an eating disorder, such as BED, and other conditions, such as depressive or anxiety disorders, substance use disorders, or disorders where impulsivity may be prominent (e.g., personality disorders). It is useful to review the patient's typical coping skills, with special attention to whether food is utilized by the individual to manage stress.

Referral to a nutritionist for food plans and further education about healthy food options is often helpful. Structured weight loss programs that include support and guidance, such as Weight Watchers, may be particularly effective for some. Changes in physical activity may be best achieved by starting a fitness routine with some interpersonal accountability—such as joining a team of others who walk every morning or signing up with a personal trainer. Various "diet" plans have been developed, written about and publicized—from the "Mediterranean Diet" to "The Zone Diet", etc. Similarly, available information on exercise regimens is just as plentiful (and potentially just as confusing to interpret), from "Cross-Fit," to Zumba, to Pilates, to marathon training. An individualized treatment plan that meets a person's needs (available time, financial resources, and personal preference, among other factors) will have the best chance of bringing not only results, but *lasting* result. Studies indicate that a large percent of overweight and obese individuals who lose weight will go on to regain the weight. Therefore, developing a plan that the individual can stick to for the long term, and adjust as needed, should be a priority. Information for patients and providers on lifestyle changes to promote healthy weight loss and weight maintenance can be found on the Web sites for the WHO, the Center for Disease Control and Prevention, and the National Institutes of Health [see References and Suggested Readings].

Addressing any comorbid psychiatric diagnoses that may be contributing to the weight issues, such as Lisa's anxiety disorder, is an important part of the comprehensive management of a case like this. Beyond addressing specific psychiatric diagnoses, it is also

important to help the individual develop improved emotional and cognitive resources—to both minimize problematic behavior that contributes to weight gain and to aid in promoting weight loss. For the person who copes with stress by eating (emotional eating), it is useful to point out this fact and then to help the individual find alternate coping strategies. Tools such as relaxation training, mindful eating, and taking a "time out" of 5 min before eating an extra serving or a "forbidden" item can help empower the person to take charge of his or her eating and to feel better equipped to handle the challenging course of weight loss and behavior change.

For some individuals, changes in lifestyle factors may not be sufficient to bring about adequate or lasting weight loss. Many "weight loss drugs" have been developed over the years, some with significant health consequences (such as the fatal cardiopulmonary side effects associated with fenfluramine/phentermine). Newer agents may have a safer side effect profile and work through a variety of mechanisms with the end result of reduced food intake [1]. These may be considered to augment changes in diet and exercise if results remain inadequate. Bariatric surgery has consistently demonstrated the most significant benefit—short- and long-term—on weight loss of all available treatments (including lifestyle changes and pharmacotherapy), but is highly invasive, with potential medical and surgical risks that render it not a first-line treatment.

For individuals with psychotropic medication-induced weight gain, there may be a role for the psychiatrist to intervene. Reviewing the patient's current eating and exercise habits, giving some general counseling, and referring to appropriate resources (online resources, weight loss programs, nutrition, primary care), as well as assessing whether there are options to reduce the doses of the implicated medications or switching to more weight-neutral medications, would be appropriate first steps. There is a literature that appears to support the addition of metformin and perhaps topiramate for antipsychotic medication-induced weight gain in cases where efforts to reduce weight through diet and exercise have not been sufficient. Metformin may be associated with nausea, an unpleasant taste in the mouth, metabolic acidosis, and even kidney injury, though is generally considered to be well-tolerated by patients. Topiramate may contribute to cognitive sluggishness and other neurological effects (dizziness, abnormal sensations),

diarrhea, and kidney stones. The psychiatrist might choose to work closely with the patient's primary care doctor when considering such interventions if there are any concerns about potentially serious side effects or medical contraindications.

12.3 Differential Diagnosis

Lisa does not fulfill criteria for a feeding and eating disorder. Nonetheless, it would be important to fully screen for a feeding and eating disorder that could be contributing to her weight gain, such as BED. Individuals with bulimia nervosa may also be overweight or even obese if their calorie intake significantly exceeds the compensatory behaviors they engage in, such as vomiting. Lisa carries a diagnosis of generalized anxiety disorder; this diagnosis can be clarified by reviewing her anxiety and related symptoms. Other psychiatric issues that may be associated with weight gain, such as excessive alcohol use in an alcohol use disorder, might be considered if there are other clues leading in this direction. Medical disorders that may contribute to weight gain or impair weight loss, such as hypothyroidism, should also be considered.

12.4 Outcome

Dr. Munn obtained a more detailed eating and physical activity history from Lisa during their next appointment. It became clear that Lisa tends to eat more (specifically, more highly palatable, processed foods, such as fast food burgers and high-calorie blended coffee drinks) when she is experiencing stress. Lisa was able to acknowledge that it becomes a "vicious cycle" for her, in which stress leads to eating more, then weight gain, which in turn makes her less likely to want to be physically active, which then impacts her energy and mood and self-esteem. She consistently denied any inappropriate compensatory behaviors to lose weight. She admitted to more substantial body image concerns—reflecting on always feeling "self-conscious" about her body and never feeling like she could truly be considered "attractive." She had never been very

athletic and described feeling "intimidated" by gyms. She also demonstrated limited knowledge about the relative nutritional value of food choices. She stated, nonetheless, that she wanted to "take charge" of her health, especially after going to her primary care doctor and finding out she was "prediabetic." With the motivation of becoming a healthier "role model" for her children, she agreed to see a nutritionist. She began preparing more food at home and being more mindful of her food choices. She joined morning group walks with other mothers in her neighborhood. She subsequently joined a gym and began strength-training and more aerobic activity. Six months later, she had lost 25 lb and had signed up for a two-day charity walk. She was engaging in more physical activities with her children. Her cholesterol, fasting glucose, and blood pressure were all within normal limits. Most importantly—she would say—she felt proud of herself and proud of what her strong body could accomplish.

References

1. Kang JG, Park CY. Anti-obesity drugs: a review about their effects and safety. Diabetes Metab J. 2012;36:13–25.
2. Kessler DA. The end of overeating: taking control of the insatiable American appetite. New York, NY: Rodale; 2009.
3. World Health Organization (WHO). http://www.who.int/mediacentre/factsheets/fs311/en/ [Accessed 9 October 2016].

Suggested Readings

Center for Disease Control (CDC). http://www.cdc.gov/obesity/data/adult.html [Accessed 9 October 2016].
National Institutes of Health (NIH). http://www.nhlbi.nih.gov/health/health-topics/topics/obe [Accessed 9 October 2016].

Part III
Patients who Eat in Odd Ways

Chapter 13
Mimi, the Quiet Little Girl

13.1 Case Presentation

Mimi is an 11-year-old girl in special education classes brought in to see her pediatrician by her father with a note from the school that says "child is eating paper towel in the bathroom." Dr. Newman has been Mimi's pediatrician since she was an infant. Mimi has always been a small child, but she had fallen farther below the average growth curve for height and weight since age 9. Mimi's father states he does not know what this is about and is only here because the school "tells me I have to bring her in." He states that he and Mimi's mother are not together, but he is still involved in Mimi's life. He works nights, while her mother works during the day. He reports that he had never heard that Mimi had been eating paper towel and thinks it might be a "mistake." Mimi walks home from her school on her own (4 blocks away). She is supposed to stay with her neighbor and the neighbor's children until her mother comes home at 6 p.m. Upon further questioning, Mimi's father states that he once saw her picking up wet sand from a bucket in the playground and putting it into her mouth; he told her to stop doing this. Later in the evaluation, he tells Dr. Newman that he also now recalls that during a visit with her last week, he noted that it looked like she "threw up in her mouth" a few times.

He reports that he asked her whether she was feeling sick and she said no and denied having vomited.

Mimi is very quiet in the evaluation room, mostly shaking her head "no" to the questions Dr. Newman asks; she simply looks at him when he asks her about eating paper towels at school or at home. Her examination is largely unremarkable, other than a weight that has not increased since her last well-child visit five months prior, and a sense of fullness in the epigastric area and right upper quadrant. There is no evidence of physical trauma.

13.2   Diagnosis/Assessment

Mimi may have a diagnosis of pica.

Pica is a disordered eating behavior in which individuals repeatedly eat non-nutritive substances for a duration of at least one month in a manner that is not consistent with developmental stage or a socially sanctioned practice, and not thought to be better explained by an another psychiatric disorder or medical condition [see Text Box: Pica: DSM-5 Criteria]. Thought to be more common in those with intellectual impairment or nutritional deficiencies (specifically iron), the overall prevalence of pica has not been clearly determined. Pica usually develops during childhood, though may persist into adulthood or may have onset in adulthood. Pica may present during pregnancy. Patients with pica may eat a variety of substances, including soil, paper, paint, and soap. It has been postulated that iron deficiency triggers ingestion of substances such as soil/dirt, and some studies have demonstrated iron deficiency in individuals with pica. This theory has flaws, however; low iron in these patients may be a result of the pica behavior (i.e., eating non-nutritive substances rather than food), not the cause, and the ingestion of substances that do not contain vitamins and other nutrients is not consistent with an adaptive response to a nutritionally deficient state. Patients will sometimes describe a craving for certain non-food items. Complications of pica include impaired nutrition and weight loss if the ingestion of non-food substances replaces a substantial amount of a person's usual food intake. Those patients who repeatedly ingest substances containing dangerous compounds may develop toxicity (e.g., lead toxicity in

children eating lead-based paint). Gastrointestinal problems are also common, including irritation of the gastrointestinal tract from the substance being eaten, or even frank obstruction if the substances being eaten cannot be easily passed. Of note, pica is separate from the disordered behavior of swallowing dangerous items in order to self-injure (such as razor blades and batteries). In addition, if pica symptoms are present in an individual with another major mental disorder (such as autism spectrum disorder—a group of patients in whom pica symptoms are more prevalent), the diagnosis of pica should only be made if the symptoms are considered significant enough to warrant additional clinical attention.

Pica: DSM-5 Diagnostic Criteria

1. Persistent eating of non-nutritive substances for a period of at least one month.
2. The eating of non-nutritive substances is inappropriate to the development of the individual.
3. The eating behavior is not part of a culturally supported or socially normative practice.
4. If occurring in the presence of another mental disorder (e.g., intellectual disability, autistic spectrum disorder, and schizophrenia) or a medical condition (including pregnancy), it is severe enough to warrant independent clinical attention.

Mimi's father also mentions an episode of possible regurgitation, raising the question of whether there may be a co-occurring diagnosis of rumination disorder (RD). RD is defined as the repeated regurgitation of food (either rechewed and reswallowed or spit out) that is not due to a clear physical condition inducing the regurgitation, for at least one month [see Text Box: Rumination Disorder: DSM-5 Criteria]. If the rumination behavior exists exclusively within the context of another feeding and eating disorder (i.e., anorexia nervosa [AN], bulimia nervosa [BN], binge eating disorder [BED], or avoidant restrictive food intake disorder [ARFID]), the additional diagnosis of RD should not be made, but it should be considered a symptom of the other feeding or eating disorder (e.g., a behavior related to binging and purging in BN). The diagnosis should not be made in the presence of a

clear medical cause for repeated regurgitation or vomiting. As in the diagnosis of pica, the diagnosis of RD should not be assigned if the symptoms exist in the context of another mental disorder, such as autism spectrum disorder, unless the symptoms are considered substantial enough to call for additional clinical attention. The prevalence of RD is thought to be low, but has not been clearly determined; it has been suggested that there may be a female predominance. Similar to pica, RD often presents during childhood and is perhaps more common in individuals with intellectual impairment, though it may develop during adulthood for the first time, and in otherwise well-functioning individuals. Etiological theories include that the rumination behavior serves a purpose of self-soothing, or reflects a compulsive or impulsive (reward-seeking) behavior pattern. The diagnosis involves that medical causes of repeated regurgitation have been ruled out. Physiological studies of these individuals demonstrate that the regurgitation is not preceded by retching (to distinguish it from vomiting), and there are no consistent findings of elevated intragastric pressures to explain the behavior. The complications of RD include dental and gastrointestinal problems (e.g., gastric and esophageal/pharyngeal irritation or damage, and gastroesophageal reflux), as well as weight loss and nutritional impairment (if the individual is engaging in rumination and reswallowing repeatedly in lieu of eating adequate daily calories).

Rumination Disorder: DSM-5 Criteria

1. Repeated regurgitation of food for a period of at least one month. Regurgitated food may be rechewed, reswallowed, or spit out.
2. The repeated regurgitation is not due to a medical condition (e.g., gastrointestinal condition).
3. The behavior does not occur exclusively in the course of anorexia nervosa, bulimia nervosa, binge eating disorder, or avoidant–restrictive food intake disorder.
4. If the behavior occurs within the context of another mental disorder (i.e., generalized anxiety disorder) or neurodevelopmental disorder (i.e., intellectual disability), it must be sufficiently severe to warrant independent clinical attention.

Pica and RD, along with an earlier iteration of ARFID [see Chap. 4 for further discussion], previously existed in the DSM-IV chapter "Disorders Usually First Diagnosed in Infancy, Childhood, or Adolescence," but were moved into the expanded chapter of Feeding and Eating Disorders in DSM-5 because of an increasing consensus that such disorders are better conceptualized as syndromes similar to other eating disorders, presenting at varying times across the life cycle. Little is known about both disorders, including etiology, prevalence, risk factors, and course of illness. This may be due to a dearth of research about either disorder; both are thought to be relatively uncommon and may be underdiagnosed, as individuals who exhibit these behaviors may often do so secretly or otherwise not come to clinical attention. Relocation of these disorders into the feeding and eating disorder chapter may serve to increase the clinical and research attention they receive.

Pica and RD are similar in that their diagnoses are largely based on observable behaviors only, without inference to motivation or other emotional or psychological processes; this distinguishes them from AN, BN, and BED, which include criteria related to body image, self-worth, or related distress. That does not mean that there are no psychological factors involved in the development or perpetuation of these disorders. Psychosocial stress and impaired interpersonal relationships and functioning have been associated with both disorders and—if present—must be addressed as part of their treatment.

13.2.1   Management

Treatment of both pica and RD involves a multidisciplinary approach, including medical and mental health providers as well as family and supports (where relevant). Associated medical issues or physical complications of the behaviors must be addressed. Other psychiatric diagnoses, especially other feeding and eating disorders, should be screened for and attended to, as indicated. Treatment strategies for pica and RD are largely behavioral, with emphasis on education about the disorder, as well as cessation of the eating behaviors and maintenance of remission. The behavioral treatment focuses on habit reversal through techniques such as

relaxation training, distraction, and positive reinforcement for refraining from the behavior. As mentioned above, identifying emotional stressors and interpersonal dynamics that might be contributing to persistence of symptoms, or lack of improvement from treatment, is an important element of the management of these disorders.

13.3 Differential Diagnosis

As discussed previously, the evaluation of pica and RD should involve screening for other psychiatric disorders, including other feeding and eating disorders and other mental disorders that may commonly co-occur with these symptoms (such as autism spectrum disorder, intellectual disability, or a psychotic disorder). Diagnoses of pica and RN should not be made if one of these other disorders is present and thought to be the primary cause of the symptoms in the clinician's estimation; treatment should focus on the primary condition. However, if the symptoms are thought to be worthy of independent clinical attention, despite existing in the context of a mental disorder other than another feeding and eating disorder, the additional diagnosis of pica or RN can be made. Of note, pica and RN *can* coexist and both diagnoses can be made in the same individual. The diagnoses should not be given if there is a clear medical cause for the behavior. Other medical disorders, such as Kleine–Levin syndrome, may present with symptoms similar to pica or RN and should first be ruled out before assigning one of these diagnoses.

13.4 Outcome

Dr. Newman ordered an abdominal X-ray and sent serum chemistries, including a comprehensive metabolic profile, lead levels, and a complete blood count. Mimi was found to have a microcytic anemia. Her abdominal imaging demonstrated mild gastric dilatation, without evidence of obstruction, and no foreign body. Further collateral from school indicated that Mimi's teacher had only

witnessed this behavior once, and it had not been noticed at home or at the neighbor's home. Similarly, there had not been further observation of regurgitation of vomiting. Dr. Newman did not feel that more medical workup was indicated but was concerned that Mimi was not meeting expectable weight gain goals and that iron deficiency, thought to be related to dietary factors, was present. In a follow-up visit with Mimi and both parents, further information was revealed, including increasing disputes between her parents. Her mother noted that Mimi was appearing more withdrawn in general and would occasionally have behavioral outbursts. She also admitted that she was ashamed to say that one day she was called by the neighbor that Mimi had not shown up after school and was then found alone in the local playground 10 minutes later.

Dr. Newman involved the clinic social worker and further time was spent assessing the family's needs and Mimi's current emotional symptoms and functioning. Because of concerns for depression, she was referred to see a psychiatrist.

Suggested Readings

Hartmann AS, Becker AE, Hampton C, Bryant-Waugh R. Pica and rumination disorder in DSM-5. Psychiatr Ann. 2012;42:426–30.

Kelly NR, Shank LM, Bakalar JL, Tanofsky-Kraff M. Pediatric feeding and eating disorders: current state of diagnosis and treatment. Curr Psychiatry Rep. 2014;16:446.

Chapter 14
Nilda's Food Allergies

14.1 Case Presentation

Nilda is an 18-year-old college freshman who has returned home
for her winter break from school and is brought in by her parents to
see her pediatrician, Dr. O'Shea, because of apparent weight loss
since the summer, as well as a change in eating habits and various
physical complaints. According to her parents, Nilda appears much
thinner than she did in August when she left for school. She is
eating very little at mealtimes, citing that she feels "full." While at
school, she would often complain to her parents that she was
feeling "sick to my stomach." Nilda admits to Dr. O'Shea that she
has been eating less, explaining that she feels "bloated" all the
time, so—even though she can often feel hungry—she becomes
quickly uncomfortable when eating and sometimes will skip meals
because of this. She has loose stools a few times a week. She also
complains of fatigue, and though her grades had been holding up
through midterms, she is worried about how she did on finals, as
she felt she "could not concentrate." She admits to reading a lot
about "food allergies" online and wonders if she needs to stop
eating gluten—"like, bread and cookies and stuff." She is not able
to clarify whether there are particular foods that make her feel
worse, but she says that recently, she has been mostly sticking to

© Springer International Publishing Switzerland 2017   131
J. Gordon-Elliott, *Fundamentals of Diagnosing and Treating
Eating Disorders*, DOI 10.1007/978-3-319-46065-9_14

eating green apples, "light" yogurt, and rice. She knows she has lost weight and tells Dr. O'Brien, "I'm sure I could use to lose some weight—I always feel like my gut is sticking out." She reports that she is happy in school and that she has made a few good friends, but she is worried that college is "just not for me," stating that she is afraid she will not be able to keep up the kinds of grades she got in high school. On review of systems, she reports that she went to the dentist last week and was found to have two cavities, her first cavities in her adult teeth.

Dr. O'Brien has been Nilda's doctor since infancy. Nilda was a generally healthy child, though began having frequent doctor's visits around age 8 through puberty, with vague abdominal symptoms which tended to correlate with return to school after vacations and other stressful events. Nilda saw the school counselor for a period of time during those years to work on her "anxieties." At age 14, Nilda's parents brought her in because she had begun eating less and seemed "weak and tired" all the time. Her medical evaluation at the time had been normal, and she was evaluated by a therapist for a possible eating disorder. She began eating more normally after several weeks in therapy, and this problem did not recur.

On examination, Nilda is 5'6" and 120 lb (BMI 19.4; her weight in August had been 128 lb, BMI 20.7). Her vital signs are normal. Her abdomen is soft, but she complains of mild right upper quadrant tenderness on palpation. Her examination is otherwise unremarkable.

14.2   Diagnosis/Assessment

No clear psychiatric diagnosis at this time.
   Rule out:

- medical illness or food intolerance leading to change in eating habits;
- an emerging restrictive eating disorder, such as anorexia nervosa (AN) or avoidant/restrictive food intake disorder (ARFID)
- bulimia nervosa (BN)

Cases like Nilda are seen fairly frequently in primary care settings. A combination of food- and body-related concerns in the setting of changes in diet and life stressors can pose a clinical challenge, raising suspicion of a variety of medical and psychiatric disorders. It is essential that the clinician considers a broad differential list and pursues a judicious workup, without prematurely jumping to any conclusions.

Could Nilda have a medical condition that could explain her current symptoms?

Absolutely. New gastrointestinal complaints with correlation to certain foods may be related to a food intolerance disorder. Nilda is not able to give a very careful report of which foods seem most associated with her symptoms, but intolerances or allergies to foods such as dairy, wheat, and gluten should be considered. She mentions "gluten" and bread products, which may mean that she has noticed that these foods are more likely to cause her symptoms, even if she has not been monitoring closely enough to be able to state that more convincingly. Gluten-related disorders have received a lot of attention in recent years. They are likely best separated out into 3 distinct disorders: celiac disease (CD), gluten allergy (GA), and non-celiac gluten sensitivity (NCGS). Though a comprehensive review of the pathophysiology, diagnosis and management of these disorders goes beyond the scope of this chapter, a brief review follows. CD is an immune-mediated enteropathy in which ingestion of gluten (a protein found in wheat, barley and rye) triggers an inflammatory response affecting the small bowel mucosa, leading to gastrointestinal (GI) symptoms, such as bloating, diarrhea, and weight loss, and extra-gastrointestinal symptoms, including anemia, dermatitis, and dental enamel hypoplasia. The diagnosis can be made clinically and supported by detection of serum markers of anti-endomysium immunoglobulin A (EMA IgA) and anti-tissue transglutaminase immunoglobulin A (tTG-IgA) as well as small bowel biopsy demonstrating the classic findings of intraepithelial lymphocytosis, crypt hyperplasia, and villous atrophy. Patients with CD—which may be present in 1 % of the population and can vary in severity of symptoms and age of onset or detection—find improvement in their symptoms with elimination of gluten from their diets. CD should be suspected in patients with unexplained weight loss, anemia, a family history of CD, or a personal or family

history of other autoimmune conditions, such as diabetes mellitus type 1, autoimmune thyroiditis, or psoriasis.

GA is an adaptive immune response to ingested gluten, triggering IgE-mediated histamine release. It may present similar to and, in combination with, wheat allergy. GA may present with GI symptoms similar to CD, in addition to typical systemic allergic responses involving the upper respiratory tract and skin. Elimination of gluten and wheat may be necessary in the management of this disorder, depending on the severity of the response.

NCGS is a syndrome of mixed GI and systemic symptoms that is proposed to be linked to gluten-containing proteins, in the absence of demonstrated CD or GA. Symptoms may include GI complaints similar to CD, as well as fatigue, headache, anxiety and depression, cognitive "fogginess", joint pain, and skin lesions. NCGS—which remains a controversial diagnosis in the absence of clear evidence that gluten proteins are the main trigger molecules for the symptoms—has been estimated to be several times more common than CD and may have overlap with other systemic syndromes such as fibromyalgia.

A correlation between gluten-related disorders and psychiatric conditions has been suggested, with evidence of an increase incidence of depressive disorders, anxiety disorders, autism spectrum disorder, and schizophrenia in individuals with CD and NCGS. One suggested mechanism involves cross-reactivity of the gliadin peptide with neurons, causing dysfunction in neuronal transmission; others have proposed that alterations in levels of free circulating tryptophan in CD may be related to changes in serotonin functioning.

Inflammatory bowel disease (IBD) is another medical disorder that might be considered in a patient presenting with diet-specific GI complaints and systemic symptoms. Other conditions that can present with food-related symptoms as well as behavior that might raise concern for eating disorder (including food avoidance) include gastroesophageal reflux disorder and (especially in children) eosinophilic esophagitis.

Could Nilda have an eating disorder? Again, absolutely.

She is presenting with food avoidance, calorie reduction, and weight loss. She expresses some body-related concerns, including reporting that she feels she could benefit from losing weight and

that she thinks she looks bloated. She is of an age where eating disorders can typically onset, and she has a history of what might have been an emerging eating disorder earlier in adolescence, though her behaviors were apparently corrected following rapid clinical attention.

Her symptoms of specific food items that she is avoiding could be consistent with ARFID [see Chap. 4 for further discussion]. Dr. O'Shea would want to ask more questions about what, specifically, she is concerned about with the foods she has eliminated in her diet. Is there a texture issue that bothers her? Is there a negative experience with the way certain foods feel while they are being swallowed? Are there other anxieties or beliefs related to particular food items that are leading her to avoid them? Teasing out the extent of her body dissatisfaction will also be important, as with ARFID the food restriction should not be in the service of losing weight due to concerns about body image (one way in which it is distinguished from AN).

Her symptoms could certainly be consistent with a developing case of AN [see Chap. 1 for further discussion]. She is restricting calories and beginning to lose weight. She may have body image dissatisfaction. Her history of anxiety and perfectionism (suggested by somatic symptoms at times of stress, as well as her worries about not being a top student in the bigger "pond" of college) may go along with this diagnosis, too. Further exploration of her ideas about her body, wish for thinness, and specific worries about food should be explored.

Though she is not reporting binge eating episodes or compensatory behaviors, such as vomiting or laxative use, she does report recent cavities. This might, if the suspicion is otherwise high, raise a question about BN [see Chap. 7 for further discussion], and additional exploration of her eating habits and food-related behaviors should be pursued. In this case, the dental enamel hypoplasia of CD, if she indeed has it, could explain the cavities—and not necessarily suggest BN.

The importance of differentiating between an eating disorder and a medical disorder:

Medical conditions that involve GI functioning and are mediated by certain foods can often present in ways that look deceptively like an eating disorder. It is important for the clinician evaluating a

patient like Nilda to be mindful of the possible presence of an eating disorder without allowing that concern to overshadow the appropriate investigation of a medical condition. On the other hand, patients with eating disorders may give a variety of justifications for their eating habits, including physical symptoms (which may be fabricated or may be a consequence of the eating disorder —e.g., delayed gastric emptying and bloating may present in both AN and BN; heartburn may occur in BN due to the repeated vomiting and might not indicate the presence of another medical cause for GERD). It is therefore essential to not take all medical complaints completely at face value and—if there are other reasons to suspect an eating disorder—to keep that in mind while doing a reasonable medical workup.

Clear medical disorders can be ruled out through investigations specific to the disorder (e.g., small intestine biopsy for CD). The confirmation, or absolute exclusion, of an eating disorder is not as easy. No laboratory findings are diagnostic of an eating disorder. In individuals with AN and BN, abnormal electrolytes may be found. Anemia is less common in eating disorders than in other medical conditions, even with significant food restriction and weight loss; normal hemoglobin, hematocrit, and ferritin levels might therefore, along with other supporting evidence from the history and physical exam, point more toward AN than an underlying medical condition (e.g., celiac disease).

The importance of not overlooking either an eating disorder or a medical disorder:

As essential as it is to not let the suspicion of a medical disorder or an eating disorder obscure the detection of the other, it is perhaps even more important to not let the diagnosis of one rule out the presence of another. In fact, eating disorders can commonly coexist with many medical disorders, perhaps especially those conditions that are related to the GI system. For example, a patient with CD with a vulnerability toward developing an eating disorder may—due to the necessary food restrictions she must follow for her CD—become increasingly preoccupied with food and how food makes her body feel; over time, symptoms of restriction beyond what is necessary for her CD might develop, with increased body image disturbances, resulting in full-criteria AN. Or a patient with CD might purposefully eat gluten-containing foods to induce "purging" through diarrhea.

From the other side of things, an eating disorder may, similarly, cause GI issues that can develop into chronic medical conditions. BN, for example, may result in disordered GI motility issues, GERD, or more serious conditions (e.g., esophageal tears). It is important, when there is suspicion of both eating disorder symptoms and a medical condition, to investigate both, with appreciation for how they might influence each other, the course of illness and the treatment.

14.2.1 Management

The discussion so far has outlined, in general terms, some of the challenges of distinguishing, diagnosing, and prioritizing various medical and psychiatric disorders in presentations like Nilda's. If there is concern about an eating disorder that co-exists with a medical condition, like CD, it will be essential to address both in a thoughtful manner. An interdisciplinary approach in which gastroenterology, mental health, and nutrition providers are collaborating and presenting a unified treatment approach will be essential, as cases with overlapping disorders can commonly lead to split opinions and recommendations that can confuse the patient or perpetuate symptoms. For example, a patient with AN and CD will have to follow a rigid gluten-free diet, but if the gastroenterology specialists are not sensitive to her AN symptoms, an overly dogmatic presentation of diet requirements may worsen her eating symptoms (e.g., if gluten-containing foods are represented as "bad," this might contribute to her distorted thoughts about food and her body); alternatively, if the mental health providers are not adequately cooperating with gastroenterology, they might recommend too much flexibility in diet (in an effort to help her expand her diet choices and break down habits of rigidity related to eating), including misguidedly encouraging her to eat gluten-containing foods. Ideally, a flexible but medically sound treatment plan can be established to allow for improvement in her eating habits while not jeopardizing her management of her medical illness. Similar principles would apply in other cases where medical and eating disorders coexist [see Chap. 6 for the discussion of eating symptoms in the context of diabetes mellitus].

When an eating disorder is suspected despite a patient's intent focus on physical symptoms and on having a medical disorder (e.g., a poorly defined food intolerance issue that the clinician, in good faith, has evaluated and determined to be highly unlikely), it is important to actively address the eating disorder while maintaining sensitivity and engaging the patient from a shared perspective. For example, if a patient with AN—after appropriate evaluation and judicious workup if indicated—is determined to be citing specific food intolerances to rationalize extreme food restriction, the clinician should clearly communicate to the patient that there is concern that an eating disorder is present and needs treatment, while avoiding aggressively refuting the presence of the food intolerance, as this may only result in alienating the patient. The clinician can validate that the patient is experiencing certain foods as adverse, while reinforcing that systematic reestablishment of a balanced, healthy diet will be essential for health and may—in fact—improve some of the physical symptoms and concerns that the patient believes to be related to those food items. Such cases can be very complicated to treat, and engagement of the patient can be extremely challenging; an interdisciplinary approach with firm but sensitive expectations about the treatment plan may help to maintain the patient's cooperation while addressing the patient's health, which might be critically at risk because of eating-related behavior.

14.3 Differential Diagnosis

As discussed previously, the differential diagnosis for Nilda is broad, including a variety of medical conditions and eating disorders. The clinician would also want to consider other psychiatric conditions, such as an anxiety disorder (e.g., she has a history of physical symptoms in the setting of stressful life events and times of separation, perhaps indicating separation anxiety disorder). In addition, the clinician would benefit from knowing about various syndromes with controversial evidence, the "prevalence" of which tend to ebb and flow depending on popular beliefs and media attention, that can present with emotional and food-related concerns. For example, there has been recent increased interest in systemic overgrowth of candida albicans (the disorder often

colloquially being referred to as "Candida"), presenting with a variety of symptoms from food malabsorption and intolerance issues, to depression, anxiety, and cognitive symptoms. There is no clear consensus on the physiologic validity of this condition, with disagreement among healthcare providers and experts, with some refuting its validity and others proposing that it is an underdiagnosed cause of numerous physical and emotional disorders. A significant amount of attention and research has also recently been emerging related to the gut microbiome and how changes in the intestinal bacterial composition may influence every body system, including mental health. A host of "fad" conditions continually appear on the Internet and in other media, with varying levels of real "science" to support the validity, efficacy, and safety of the "treatments" being offered. A patient with an eating disorder might be particularly susceptible to latching onto one of these disorders that are professed to be related to certain food items, and the treatment of which require elimination of those foods. A "medical reason" to avoid certain foods or restrict one's diet can be used to obfuscate or otherwise perpetuate an eating disorder. These clinical scenarios can be very complicated to assess and tease out, especially when the medical condition being cited is less clearly defined or less straightforward to confirm by usual diagnostic strategies.

14.4 Outcome

Dr. O'Shea had concern for CD when meeting with Nilda, and—in fact—the workup confirmed the diagnosis. Nilda began a gluten-free diet, which improved many of her physical symptoms. Unfortunately, despite these improvements, rigidity around diet and overall calorie restriction was still being observed by her parents. Further exploration of her ideas about her body and food raised concerns for symptoms of emerging AN. Nilda, for example, was refusing gluten-free baked goods, despite education on how these should not perpetuate her physical symptoms; and she would occasionally make off-hand comments about feeling "unattractive" and wanting to "tone up." She was referred to see a therapist and continued to work with her over the next several months, having decided to take a medical leave from school. With time, Nilda was

able to express more deeply held negative ideas about her body, and her wish to make her body "so small I don't get noticed." A few depressive symptoms were noted, but in consultation with a psychiatrist, it was decided that further psychotherapy, addressing her eating symptoms, would be an appropriate initial treatment plan. A behavioral program was instituted, reintroducing a wider range of food into her diet and engaging her in pleasurable activities involving food (such as enjoyable outings with friends and family where a meal was part of the agenda), to desensitize her to her negative experience of eating. Nilda progressively became less preoccupied with food items, and despite gaining back some of the weight she had been losing (stabilizing at 123 lb), she was noted to be less concerned about her body and to take more pride in her body and appearance. Her depressive symptoms also improved. She was able to take a course at the local community college that summer and then returned to college in the fall. She maintained her gluten-free diet, her weight stabilized, and she had a successful year, academically and socially.

Suggested Readings

Allen PJ. Gluten-related disorders: celiac disease, gluten allergy, non-celiac gluten sensitivity. Pediatr Nurs. 2015;41:146–50.

Bern EM, O'Brien RF. Is it an eating disorder, gastrointestinal disorder, or both? Curr Opin Pediatr. 2013;25:463–70.

Jackson JR, Eaton WW, Cascella NG, Fasano A, Kelly DL. Neurologic and psychiatric manifestations of celiac disease and gluten sensitivity. Psychiatr Q. 2012;83:91–102.

Chapter 15
Olive, the Healthy Eater

15.1 Case Presentation

Olive is a 68-year-old divorced woman who brings herself into the urgent care clinic complaining of "full body weakness" and "pain in my hands and feet." She explains that for the past three years, she has become aware of numerous "environmental allergens" that she is being exposed to, such as "toxic chemicals" in the air in the hallways of her building, and "impure foods" at restaurants and supermarkets. She has been participating in online chat rooms about toxic environmental exposures and has been following an "elimination diet" prescribed by one of the "experts" she found online. She reports that she gets her food at her local health food store and that her diet currently consists of white rice, herbal tea, and coconut water. She feels that all other foods cause her to have negative "allergic reactions." She also says that she wants to only eat food that is "healthy and pure" and spends hours reading and comparing the ingredient lists of other food items in the store. She admits that she is "quite thin" and denies wanting to lose weight. She complains of feeling like her legs are weak and that she has been dropping things from her hands; in addition, she describes burning pain in her hands and feet.

© Springer International Publishing Switzerland 2017
J. Gordon-Elliott, *Fundamentals of Diagnosing and Treating Eating Disorders*, DOI 10.1007/978-3-319-46065-9_15

Olive is 5'3" and weighs 95 lb (BMI 16.8). She appears very thin with evidence of temporal wasting. She is somewhat unkempt, with long hair in a loose braid, and ungroomed fingernails; her clothes appear too large for her body. She is alert and attentive. Her heart rate is regular though with two skipped beats over a 60 second period. Her blood pressure is 95/70 mm Hg without orthostatic changes. Subtle horizontal nystagmus is noted bilaterally, and her strength in her major motor groups is decreased (4+/5). The rest of her exam is unremarkable. An electrocardiogram shows sinus rhythm at 58 beats per minute, with occasional premature ventricular contractions (PVCs). Laboratory studies demonstrate a macrocytic anemia, with low potassium, magnesium, albumin, and vitamin B12 level; thyroid-stimulating hormone is at the upper limit of normal, but free thyroxine is normal; creatinine and blood urea nitrogen are both just above normal limits; blood alcohol level is undetectable.

15.2   Diagnosis/Assessment

Vitamin B12 deficiency has been demonstrated. Olive's presentation may be consistent with a broad range of other medical and psychiatric conditions and requires further evaluation. Olive is presenting with low weight (and suspected weight loss, given her oversized clothes), specific and idiosyncratic beliefs and behaviors related to eating, and medical/neurologic abnormalities. Given her age, and physical exam and laboratory findings, a further medical work-up is essential.

Vitamin B12 deficiency may explain the macrocytic anemia, muscle weakness, and paresthesias. Vitamin B12 deficiency can be due to limited dietary intake (most common in vegan diets, which eliminate all animal products, as well as other highly restricted diets) or impaired absorption (e.g., due to changes in stomach and small bowel functioning, deficient intrinsic factor, or immune disorders such as Grave's disease or lupus). It may present with anemia with elevated mean corpuscular volume, gastrointestinal symptoms, and neurologic findings, including abnormalities of reflexes, sensation, and strength, as well as fatigue, cognitive impairment, and psychiatric syndromes (e.g., mania, psychosis).

Methylmalonic acid and homocysteine levels may be elevated. Olive's restricted diet has likely caused her to be vitamin B12 deficient.

The clinician might be considering additional vitamin deficiencies, including vitamin B1 (thiamine), which may cause muscle weakness and atrophy, hypotension, heart failure, neurologic findings, and mental status changes. Wernicke's encephalopathy, which classically has been associated with alcohol use but can develop in any individual with thiamine deficiency, is comprised of ophthalmoplegia, ataxia, and confusion. Impaired intake of thiamine deficiency occurs in restricted diets or general malnutrition; as many foods are fortified with thiamine, such as breads and cereal, a diet centered largely around white rice and processed foods might be more likely to lead thiamine deficiency. People who drink excessive alcohol often have impaired thiamine intake because they are largely consuming their calories through alcohol and eat poorly otherwise; in addition, alcohol may inhibit some of the necessary biochemical process required for thiamine absorption and metabolism. Thiamine deficiency may also be due to increased urinary losses in people with kidney disease.

Olive's limited diet may also be causing her electrolyte abnormalities, which may be contributing to her cardiac findings (bradycardia, PVCs) and weakness. Her diet is not only restricted in nutritional value, but also severely deficient in calories, leading to her weight loss and general evidence of malnutrition, including temporal wasting. Other medical considerations should include heavy metal toxicity, neurodegenerative conditions, gastrointestinal disorders (such as Crohn's disease), and cancer.

She's odd—she says odd things, eats oddly, and looks a little odd… could there be an underlying psychiatric component to her presentation?

Indeed, as pointed out in Chap. 14, even in the presence of a medical condition there may be psychiatric or behavioral issues that are independent, related, or contributing. A medical problem such as vitamin deficiency may lead to physical findings and psychiatric signs and symptoms. Psychiatric disturbances may, analogously, lead to changes in behavior that then contribute to the development of medical issues. In Olive's case, the evaluating clinician should absolutely be wondering whether her strange approach to diet, which subsequently may be contributing to her

medical signs and symptoms, could be a function of mental health problem. If so, what?

Eating disorders:

Olive could have an eating disorder. She is rigid about what she eats and refers to spending a substantial amount of time thinking about what she eats. She denies wanting to lose weight and she does not demonstrate clear evidence of disordered body image, but she may not be forthcoming about these things. Her presentation could be consistent with anorexia nervosa [AN, see Chap. 1 for further discussion], with food restriction for the purpose of losing weight. As discussed in Chap. 14, patients with AN may obfuscate their symptoms behind philosophies about diet or nutrition plans that they report they are following for "health" reasons, while—in fact—the diets are primarily in place for the purpose of restricting calories.

Some individuals present with very strict beliefs about food, and only eat foods that are considered wholly "healthy." Such individuals will go to great lengths to find what they believe are the "purest" foods and strive for "healthy eating," which will inevitably limit the range of acceptable foods they can eat and may lead to weight loss if not enough "healthy food" calories are consumed to maintain their energy needs. They may read books or online resources, consult health "experts" who may prescribe elimination diets or other nutritional plans, and spend hours reviewing the content of foods they might consider eating. The term *orthorexia nervosa* (from the Greek *orthos*, meaning "right" or "correct") has been proposed to describe these individuals. There is discussion about whether this presentation should be considered an eating disorder, in and of itself. Some might argue that these behaviors may only be adopted in the service of losing weight, and therefore, this syndrome would more aptly be considered a possible presentation of AN. On the other hand, it may be that individuals who eat in this way have more in common with patients with obsessive compulsive and related disorders, or somatic symptom disorders, if, instead, the disorder is conceptualized as being driven primarily by dysfunctional preoccupation with "healthy food" and the effects of "unhealthy" foods on the body. The evaluation of a patient presenting in this way requires careful assessment for comorbid psychiatric conditions, psychological processes, and personality traits; a precise appreciation of the factors underlying the behaviors

will allow for a more accurate formulation and development of an appropriate treatment plan.

Another eating disorder that could explain Olive's behavior is avoidant restrictive food intake disorder [ARFID, see Chap. 14 for further discussion]; further exploration of whether there are particular aspects of food—texture, taste, worries about what the food is doing to her body—may be useful in assessing for whether this diagnosis would explain her presentation.

Disorders involving psychotic symptoms:

Olive might have a psychotic disorder, such as schizophrenia or delusional disorder, or a depressive disorder with psychotic symptoms (i.e., major depressive disorder with psychotic features). Her beliefs about food may be psychotic in nature, with complex ideas about what constitutes "healthy" or "toxic." Patients with odd or "eccentric" personalities, such as schizotypal personality disorder, may similarly present with idiosyncratic beliefs about food, which may become more rigidly held over time.

Somatic symptom disorders:

Olive's concerns about "toxic" elements of the environment and unhealthy foods might be consistent with a somatic symptom disorder (SSD). Excessive concerns about her body and health, the food she eats, and the environment in which she lives, could be part of an SSD. Olive specifically mentions her concerns about environmental toxins and the "allergies" she experiences. The clinician might want to explore this more with her to better understand her beliefs and behaviors related to these concerns. Idiopathic environmental intolerances (IEI), a syndrome that was previously referred to as multiple chemical sensitivity (MCS), is a controversial clinical entity of multiple and varied physical symptoms that are attributed to environmental influences, such as chemicals in buildings or cleaning products, foods, or other physical exposures. The health complaints of individuals who are considered to have IEI are variable and often idiosyncratic, from physical issues such as breathing problems, to neuropsychiatric concerns such as fatigue or depression. There may be substantial overlap between these patients and individuals with SSDs, as well as fibromyalgia and chronic fatigue disorder. Some would argue that IED is just a modern-day equivalent of an entity that has existed throughout time, but with a current explanation—environmental allergens and toxins. Whereas in past eras, those with poorly explained fatigue,

emotional distress, pain, or other non-specific symptoms might have been thought to have *neurasthenia* (a condition comprising of such symptoms, commonly considered due to the stress of living in the industrialized world), some may now be attributing these same issues to IEI. With substantial disagreement about the validity of this entity, and limited clear data to support it, IEI remains a controversial diagnosis and one that many mental health experts would consider primarily a psychiatric disturbance, likely most closely related to an SSD.

Neurocognitive disorders:

Several features of Olive's presentation suggest a neurocognitive disorder, such as dementia. An older adult presenting with demonstration of deterioration in self-care and functioning should prompt the question of cognitive decline. As cognitive status, perhaps specifically executive features of cognitive functioning, becomes more impaired, individuals may begin to show signs of compromised activities of daily living. They may forget to eat or have more difficulty structuring their behavior in order to provide themselves with the food that they need (e.g., going to the store, knowing what to buy and what constitutes a healthy diet, preparing the food). These individuals may develop a much more limited diet, utilizing only a few food groups, with progressively less diversity in food options over time. The term "tea and toast diet" refers to this phenomenon that may be seen in older adults, especially as their executive cognitive functioning declines. These findings may be found in any type of dementia and may be associated with the development of related features, such as hoarding behavior or psychotic symptoms. These individuals may also experience impairment in other aspects of daily living, such as paying bills, keeping their homes and belongings tidy and in order, and engaging in productive work and social activities. A thorough evaluation would include a medical work-up for any issues that could be impairing cognition and potentially reversible (such as vitamin deficiencies, factors contributing to delirium), an assessment of cognitive functioning (e.g., a structured test such as the Montreal Cognitive Assessment [MoCA], or the Mini-Mental Status Exam [MMSE]), and additional relevant testing if indicated (e.g., brain imaging). Modifiable behaviors contributing to the cognitive impairment, such as excessive alcohol use or poor diet, would ideally be corrected A careful evaluation of the patient's

current functioning and safety should be done. Contacting family or other supports and assessing the home environment will be another important part of the assessment.

15.2.1 Eating Disorders in Older Adults

Eating disorders are generally thought of as conditions associated with young women from adolescence to early adulthood. In fact, eating disorders affect both men and women [see Chaps. 5, 9 and 10 for more discussion of eating disorders in males] and individuals across the life span. The incidence of eating disorders in older adults appears to be increasing. With demographic shifts and a larger percent of the total population in midlife and later adulthood, eating disorders in older adults will likely become more prevalent and of increasing clinical significance. AN and bulimia nervosa [BN] affect adults in midlife and beyond, though seemingly at lower rates than present in younger populations. It has been postulated that most cases of AN and BN in older adults represent chronic disorders rather than new cases first developing in midlife or later. This would be supported by the literature which indicates that the long-term prognosis of AN, for example, is guarded, with as much as one half of patients continuing to have symptoms and relapses over their lifetime. There may be an increase in new or recurrent episodes of eating disorders in the perimenopause period, perhaps due to a combination of neuroendocrine and psychological factors relevant to the end of the reproductive phase of life, analogous to the onset at puberty (when eating disorders may begin to become prevalent). Binge eating disorder [BED] is the most common specific eating disorder in older life, which correlates with its overall higher prevalence and tendency to onset or peak at a later age than AN and BN. Subsyndromal BED (binge eating episodes without the frequency or associated psychological distress to meet criteria for BED) may be particularly common in midlife, with relatively high rates in individuals in their 40s, 50s, and 60s.

Older adults with low food intake and weight loss pose a particular diagnostic problem as reviewed so far in this chapter—

namely, is this an eating disorder or something else? Indeed, as discussed above, other psychiatric and medical conditions can lead to odd or restricted eating patterns. Normal aging may also be a factor, with reduced appetite and food intake occurring commonly as individuals' age. "Anorexia of aging" may affect 20 % of older adults, with a general decline in calorie, macro-, and micronutrient intake, and may be a function of numerous factors related to aging, including alterations in taste and smell, neuroendocrine changes, and medical and psychiatric conditions. Pharmacologic treatments to increase appetite, such as megestrol acetate and dronabinol appear to have minimal benefit in such cases, though research is limited.

Eating disorders in older adults may be particularly challenging to treat given the chronic course and refractory nature of symptoms in this population. In general, individuals with eating disorders may be difficult to engage meaningfully in treatment, often seeking help temporarily for help with physical consequences of the disorders, but often dropping out of care before substantial treatment gains have been accomplished; moreover, the relapse rate is high even after initial recovery. Nonetheless, the same principles would apply to older adults with an eating disorder such as AN as with younger individuals, including medical stabilization, weight restoration, engagement in treatment to normalize eating behavior, and involvement of family and other supports. Psychopharmacologic treatments, at least for AN, have not been found to have robust utility, though judicious use of antidepressants or antipsychotics may help when there are co-occurring symptoms of depression or anxiety [see Chap. 1 for further discussion of the management of AN].

The medical, emotional, and social consequences of eating disorders are substantial and as relevant in older adults as they are in younger patients. Reduced bone density from calorie restriction in AN is of particular importance in older adults who have an increased rate of osteopenia, osteoporosis and bone fractures. Pharmacologic management, including bisphosphonates and estrogen replacement, have uncertain benefit in this population. Older adults with AN and BN appear to be less likely than individuals without these disorders to be married and have children, perhaps indicating an effect of these conditions on interpersonal functioning with lasting impact.

15.2.2 Treatment

Management of a patient with a presentation like Olive's will depend upon the underlying issue or issues. First and foremost, any treatable or reversible medical conditions should be addressed. After stabilization of vitamin deficiencies, endocrinopathies, alcohol use, or other contributing factors, an evaluation of comorbid psychiatric disorders, and development of a targeted treatment plan, can then be done.

Patients like Olive, because of the complexity of medical, psychiatric, and social issues at play, usually require a multidisciplinary approach—involving medical and mental health clinicians, nursing, and social services. The patient may need more supervision at home, or even transition to a more supervised setting. Family or other supports may need to become involved; in those cases where significant cognitive impairment is present, a surrogate may be obliged to take responsibility for financial, legal, and healthcare decision making.

15.3 Differential Diagnosis

As reviewed in detail above, a patient like Olive will prompt consideration of numerous different and potentially overlapping disorders, including a range of medical and psychiatric conditions. An eating disorder, potentially comorbid with, or contributing to, the rest of the clinical picture, may be identified. In cases like this, it is important to not miss the presence of an eating disorder, but—just as important—to not fall into the trap of attributing all problems to an eating disorder; keeping an open mind, considering the full differential diagnosis, and addressing the patient's problem list in a rigorous and stepwise fashion will allow for provision of the best possible care.

15.4   Outcome

Olive was admitted to the hospital. Her vitamin B12 was repleted
with parenteral supplementation. Vitamin B1 deficiency, subsequently revealed, was addressed with high-dose intravenous thiamine. She scored 18/30 on the MoCA, demonstrating moderate
cognitive impairment. Her niece was contacted who visited her
apartment, finding it to be in significant disarray. There was no
evidence of alcohol in the home. Upon further questioning, her
niece indicated that—though her aunt had always lived a fairly
"solitary" life, she and the rest of the family were aware that Olive
had always been thin and preoccupied with her eating and weight.
She had, in fact, been admitted to an eating disorder inpatient
program 30 years prior. After three weeks in the hospital, with
improved nutrition, Olive was noted to be less preoccupied with
her food choices and was able to begin eating a more varied diet.
She, unfortunately, continued to do poorly on evaluation of executive functioning and there was significant concern about her
ability to manage safely at home. Her niece authorized transfer to a
physical rehabilitation facility, with the plan to proceed with
transitioning her to a supervised residential setting.

Suggested Readings

Finney GR, Minagar A, Heilman KM. Assessment of mental status. Neurol
    Clin. 2016;34:1–16.
Koven NS, Abry AW. The clinical basis of orthorexia nervosa: emerging
    perspectives. Neuropsychiatr Dis Treat. 2015;11:385–94.
Mangweth-Matzek B, Hoek HW, Pope HG Jr. Pathological eating and body
    dissatisfaction in middle-aged and older women. Curr Opin Psychiatry.
    2014;27:431–5.
Podfigurna-Stopa A, Czyzyk A, Katulski K, Smolarczyk, Grymowicz M,
    Maciejewska-Jeske M, Meczekalski B. Eating disorders in older women.
    Maturitas. 2015;82:146–152.

Chapter 16
Peter, Healthy Weight but Unhealthy

16.1 Case Presentation

Peter is a 24-year-old single man, living in low-income housing with his grandmother, working at a local chain drug store/pharmacy, who is coming to see Dr. Quinn for the first time for a checkup and refill of his asthma inhalers. Peter admits that he has not been to a doctor for "a few years." He reports that he was treated for asthma as a child but felt he had "grown out of it"; recently, he began playing pickup games of basketball and had an asthma attack during a game last week, prompting this visit. Peter denies having any other medical issues and has no additional physical complaints. He takes no medicines. He reports occasional alcohol use, drinking "a six-pack" once a week, on average, when hanging out with friends; he denies daily use and denies that his drinking has a negative impact on his work or social functioning. He denies tobacco or cannabis use, acknowledging that when he has smoked in the past it has led to asthma symptoms. He denies any other substance use. He denies any mental health symptoms. Peter reports working five days a week at the drug store, the 4 pm–midnight shift, stocking shelves. When he leaves work, he tends to go to the local fast food restaurant where he picks up a meal. His lunch is usually also fast food. He will sometimes eat a roll with

© Springer International Publishing Switzerland 2017
J. Gordon-Elliott, *Fundamentals of Diagnosing and Treating Eating Disorders*, DOI 10.1007/978-3-319-46065-9_16

butter on his way to work, or he will skip this first meal of the day. He has not been getting regular exercise since high school, when he played on his school's basketball team, but, as noted, he has recently started playing again. He denies any recent changes in weight and states that he has never been overweight. He says that he does not make enough money in his job to live on his own at this point and has chosen to stay with his grandmother, who has been living in her subsidized rental for 40 years. She is 62 years old and Peter worries about her, because she has been having more health problems; her son (Peter's father) had been her main support, but he has recently been unable to care for her as he had a stroke at age 43. Peter has not had much contact with his father, but says that he is "heavy-set" and also may have "done some drugs".

On exam, Peter is a trim young man, appearing well. His heart rate is 72, blood pressure is 132/70, height is 6′3″, and weight is 180 lb (BMI 22.5). His heart and lung exam is unremarkable. Dr. Quinn refers him for pulmonary function tests and suggests that they check his cholesterol and sugar levels. She also asks him if he would like to talk more about his diet, as she thinks that with a few changes in his nutrition (such as reduced sodium intake) his elevated systolic blood pressure might improve. She explains that he might be at increased risk for things such as diabetes, heart attack, and stroke in the future—acknowledging his grandmother's and father's health issues—and that he could help decrease his risk factors with some adjustments in what he eats and how he takes care of himself. Peter says he has in fact been wondering about this recently and would be interested in learning more.

16.2 Diagnosis/Assessment

No feeding and eating disorder diagnosis. Rule out alcohol use disorder.

Peter does not have an eating disorder. He has no identified preoccupations with food or his body, and his eating is not clearly causing any impairment in his general functioning. Nonetheless, Peter eats in ways that put him at risk for malnutrition and chronic disease.

Food security has been defined by the World Food Summit as the state of having reliable "access to sufficient, safe, nutritious food to maintain a healthy and active life." In 2014, 15 % of households in the USA were food insecure at some point. In addition to basic food safety and hygiene, the main factors involved in food security are availability and access. Low-income individuals are more likely than those of higher socioeconomic status to have limited access to healthful foods, and to live in so-called *food deserts*—areas with scarce available fruits and vegetables and other healthful whole foods as would be found in grocery stores and farmers' markets. Individuals living in areas like these may more commonly purchase food in convenience stores, where food prices are typically higher than in larger supermarkets. Healthy food options, especially affordable ones, will be limited in such settings. Fast food restaurants' pricing system may promote the purchase of unhealthy items because such items may include a higher amount of calories per dollar spent—thus offering a cost advantage, which is especially relevant for individuals with limited money available to pay for food. For these reasons, among others, individuals from low socioeconomic backgrounds may be more susceptible to poor quality diets, even when knowledge about nutrition is adequate.

Overweight and obesity, distinct from eating disorders, per se, but influenced by eating habits and food availability, have become an increasing concern in this country and the world, with two-thirds of the US population currently in the overweight range (BMI 25–29.9), and a full one-third of the country in the obese range (BMI > 30). The socioeconomic and cultural influences of weight are complex and not straightforward. While limited access to healthy foods and more unhealthful eating practices might be associated with development of weight issues, obesity does not appear to be clearly associated with race, ethnicity, or socioeconomic status, at least when evaluated across racial/ethnic, education, and gender divisions.

Eating disorders and food security are separate issues, and yet to some extent interrelated. Historically, it has been thought that eating disorders—or, at least, the prototypical disorders of anorexia nervosa (AN) and bulimia nervosa (BN)—are problems afflicting those of privileged backgrounds, thus largely affecting high-income, Caucasian individuals. This notion is not accurate,

with eating disorders impacting individuals across all racial/ethnic and socioeconomic groups; this applies, too, across gender, sexuality, and educational level. Studies indicate an increase in eating disordered behavior, including binge eating and compensatory behaviors, as well as negative body image, in non-white racial groups and in men over the past 20 years. Theories about certain racial and ethnic minority groups being relatively "immune" to eating disorders, perhaps because of alternate beauty standards within their communities, have been largely debunked. Moreover, groups with higher prevalence of obesity may exhibit thoughts, attitudes, and behaviors of disordered eating; the presence of eating disorders in such groups should not be overlooked.

Peter does not have an eating disorder and is of normal weight. He has elevated blood pressure, which may be related to sodium intake or other aspects of his current diet. He eats foods with an unhealthy composition of cholesterol, fat, sugar, and highly processed ingredients. His diet may put him at increased risk for developing cardiovascular and cerebrovascular disease, kidney disease, cancer and diabetes, among other chronic conditions. Diet, in addition to activity level, body mass, and tobacco smoking, is considered a modifiable risk factor for developing chronic disease. Peter would benefit from adopting a more balanced diet and from continuing to engage in regular exercise, which he has recently been beginning to do. Studies show that it is not just education about diet and access to healthy foods that allow for better food choices, but that cost of healthful food options is a major factor. Clinicians may not be able to control the price or availability of food options for their patients, but it is reasonable to assume that counseling about dietary guidelines and exercise can have some impact on patients' behaviors. Awareness of local programs that enhance the availability and affordability of healthful food may allow the clinician to offer useful suggestions to patients.

Peter seems to be receptive to information at this time—perhaps specifically because of growing concerns he has been having about his health due to family health issues. This offers the clinician an excellent opportunity to counsel him, validating his concerns and helping him to see that he may have options for modifying his own health destiny. Dr. Quinn can explore with Peter the aspects of his life that influence his dietary and exercise habits, including his schedule and finances. Together, they can explore ways for him to

make small changes that may have a positive impact on his health, including better food choices and other lifestyle adjustments. A nutritional consultation and information about resources available to him in his community (for healthful food and exercise) might bring additional benefit. Information for patients and providers on lifestyle changes to promote healthy weight loss and weight maintenance can be found on the websites for the World Health Organization, the Center for Disease Control and Prevention, and the National Institutes of Health [see Chap. 12 for more information and references]. If nothing else, talking openly with Peter about the impact that he could potentially have in improving his health, and maintaining good health in the future, could empower him and give him an increased sense of self-esteem.

16.3   Differential Diagnosis

There are no identified signs of a feeding and eating disorder in Peter's presentation. As stated above, individuals across ethnicity, race, gender, socioeconomic, and educational lines should be screened for eating disorders when suspected. It is essential that clinicians be observant for any eating- and body-related symptoms in all individuals, regardless of background, lest eating disorder pathology be missed and not addressed.

16.4   Outcome

Dr. Quinn gave Peter positive feedback about his wanting to know more about what he can do to improve his health and stay healthy in the future. She encouraged his recent efforts to increase his physical activity. She agreed that his family history is concerning and could be a reason for him to attend even more closely to his health. She asked him to talk with her about what he knows about healthy nutrition and exercise and how these impact medical issues and the development of chronic diseases. She had him go through in more detail how he structures his day and ways in which he might be able to make small adjustments in his behaviors and food

choices to optimize his health. She spoke with him about sleep hygiene. She also explored his use of alcohol and counseled him about the recommended amount of alcohol for men his age, as well as screened him for concerning signs of an alcohol use disorder (the CAGE screening tool [see NIAAA link in Suggested Readings for more information]). Dr. Quinn asked Peter if he would be interested in seeing the nutritionist in the clinic for further information about his dietary choices. She also involved the clinic social worker for additional information about resources in the community for accessing healthful foods for Peter and his grandmother.

Suggested Readings

Coleman-Jensen A, Rabbitt MP, Gregory C, Singh A. Household food security in the United States in 2014. United States Department of Agriculture Economic Research Service: Economic Research Report, Number 194 (September 2015). Found at: http://www.ers.usda.gov/media/1896841/err194.pdf

Franklin B, Jones A, Love D, Puckett S, Macklin J, White-Means S. Exploring mediators of food insecurity and obesity: a review of recent literature. J Community Health. 2012;37:253–64.

Mitchison D, Hay P, Slewa-Younan S, Mond J. The changing demographic profile of eating disorder behaviors in the community. BMC Public Health. 2014;14:943.

National Institute of Alcohol Abuse and Alcoholism (NIAAA). http://pubs.niaaa.nih.gov/publications/arh28-2/78-79.htm [Accessed 9 October 2016].

Ogden CL, Lamb MM, Carroll MD, Flegal KM. Obesity and socioeconomic status in adults: United States, 2005–2008. National Center for Health Statistics Data Brief, Number 50 (December 2010). Found at: http://www.cdc.gov/nchs/data/databriefs/db50.pdf

Index

© Springer International Publishing Switzerland 2017
J. Gordon-Elliott, *Fundamentals of Diagnosing and Treating
Eating Disorders*, DOI 10.1007/978-3-319-46065-9

Printed in the United States
By Bookmasters